Praise for *Pain Erasers*

T0023277

"At *Woman's World* and *First for Women*, our teams have been relying on Michelle Schoffro Cook's natural healing wisdom for more than a decade. We've come to expect the very best advice grounded simultaneously in time-tested folk practices and the latest science. And yet even with those high expectations, I was surprised at the power and practicality of her newest book *Pain Erasers*.

Schoffro Cook explores 20 natural pain remedies—some very well-known and others surprising—first putting them in cultural and historical context, then exploring the science that supports their benefits and finally giving highly practical advice related to making them work in the real world. Using personal experience and extensive knowledge of supporting pain remedies, she creates a comprehensive resource I can see myself turning to again and again. If you suffer from any kind of pain, you want to get your hands on this book—and the sooner the better!"

—Carol Brooks, editorial director of
Woman's World and *First for Women*

"Yes! It *is* possible to reclaim an active, vibrant life—Dr. Michelle Schoffro Cook speaks from personal experience, having found the solutions that helped her manage her own debilitating pain. *Pain Erasers* arms readers with the latest science and effective strategies that can help mitigate pain. From an exploration of time-tested remedies to a cutting-edge look at the gut-pain theory, this comprehensive guide illustrates how to set the foundation for a healthy, pain-free body for life. *Pain Erasers* offers a wealth of information for the millions battling chronic pain—and for their doctors, too."

—Maggie Jaqua, editor-in-chief of
WholeFoods Magazine

PAIN ERASERS

Also by Michelle Schoffro Cook

Essential Oils for Hormone Bliss
The Essential Oils Healing Deck
Be Your Own Herbalist
The Cultured Cook
60 Seconds to Slim
The Ultimate pH Solution
Arthritis-Proof Your Life
Allergy-Proof Your Life
Boost Your Brain Power in 60 Seconds
The Probiotic Promise
Weekend Wonder Detox

PAIN ERASERS

The Complete Natural Medicine Guide to Safe, Drug-Free Relief

MICHELLE SCHOFFRO COOK, PhD, DNM

BenBella Books, Inc.
Dallas, TX

BenBella Books, Inc.
10440 N. Central Expressway
Suite 800
Dallas, TX 75231
www.benbellabooks.com
Send feedback to feedback@benbellabooks.com

BenBella is a federally registered trademark.

Printed in the United States of America
10 9 8 7 6 5 4 3 2 1

Library of Congress Control Number: 2021012412
ISBN 9781953295514
ebk ISBN 9781953295859

Copyediting by Jennifer Greenstein
Proofreading by Jenny Bridges and Sarah Vostok
Indexing by Amy Murphy
Text design and composition by PerfecType, Nashville, TN
Cover design by Oceana Garceau
Cover photography by Shutterstock
Printed by Lake Book Manufacturing

Special discounts for bulk sales are available. Please contact bulkorders@benbellabooks.com.

To my dear friend Dr. Robert Laquerre, DC, for your compassionate healing, the instrumental role you played in helping me to overcome severe pain, as well as for your friendship, which I value immensely

CONTENTS

Part 3: Living a Pain-Free Life

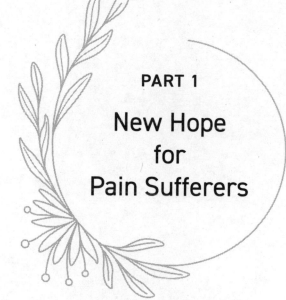

PART 1

New Hope for Pain Sufferers

INTRODUCTION

I know pain. I know the aching, throbbing, arthritic kind. I'm familiar with the bruised and burning, torn muscles variety. I know the shooting, knifing, excruciating pain of migraines, nerve damage, and body injuries. Whatever pain's expression, I'm familiar with its work. I suffered a severe car accident that left me with a partially severed spinal cord. The emergency room physician told me I was *this* close to being quadriplegic. As if that was not enough, I later experienced the unbearable agony of a broken back.

I felt constant and severe pain for many years. It nearly destroyed my life. My pain was so debilitating that I found it almost impossible to work, perform normal day-to-day functions, or have much of a life. I tried everything to which I was introduced but nothing worked well or lasted long. Pain medications should have been a welcome respite, but even prescription narcotics offered no noticeable relief. And since they were highly addictive and replete with terrible side effects, I stopped using them within a week of receiving the prescription more than twenty years ago.

On one particular occasion, I had stayed indoors, alone in the darkness of my bedroom, away from all light and noise, suffering with a migraine for nearly a week. This was a common occurrence and had been a significant part of my life for the past several years. On this day, like many others, I was desperate for the pain to end and feeling despondent that it would never be over. Eventually, I balanced my desire to race toward a solution with my need to step gingerly to avoid exacerbating the pain and headed downstairs. I wanted to look up possible emergency services. It was nearly six o'clock on a Saturday evening. My husband exclaimed, "Nothing will be open."

Tears running down my eyes, I knew he was right. But I needed help. I found an emergency hotline answered by a compassionate doctor, who after asking me a series of questions, advised me to come straight to his clinic. This doctor of chiropractic spent two hours running tests and X-rays, conducting manual mobility and spinal cord assessments, and showing me the various problems in my spinal cord, nerves, and more, which were contributing to my pain. The doctor didn't stop there. He explained various natural remedies, treatments, and exercises I could do to alleviate the pain. And he asked my husband if he would be willing to assist, which of course he was. So Dr. Robert Laquerre, this compassionate doctor whom I am fortunate to now call a dear friend, taught my husband additional ways to help me relieve pain.

I left Dr. Rob's clinic feeling lighter, with a significant reduction in pain and a sense of freedom I hadn't known in years. I could barely hold myself together as we went back to the car. The moment I sat down, I began sobbing—this time with tears of joy. I was overwhelmed with relief that the pain had finally dissipated. Perhaps, even greater than my pleasure over the elimination of the pain was the empowerment I felt because I finally had some solutions to help me deal with the pain whenever it might return, which, given the severity of the causes of my pain, it did indeed.

But, for the first time, I had some effective pain management options, and now that I had periods without pain, or with much less pain, I was able to look deeper into the remedies Dr. Rob suggested. As I continuously improved, I was able to spend more time trying to discover other natural remedies that might help me.

Motivated by my progress and hoping to permanently end the excruciating pain that had become my life for so many years, I spent hours and hours reading up on proven natural painkillers. Before meeting Dr. Rob and starting my research, I believed that nothing in nature could be as potent as drugs, but my desperation forced me to give natural options a fair chance. And my experiences and research proved me wrong: I discovered that many of the most powerful anti-pain remedies are found in nature in the form of herbs, essential oils, and nutrients.

The problem with most natural options, however, is that they rarely come with adequate instructions on their effective use. I don't think the manufacturers intend to leave people in the dark on the best ways to use their products, but most producers of natural medicines are limited in the claims or guidance they can give customers due to legal restrictions placed upon them by regulatory authorities.

I began using my body as a laboratory, experimenting with a wide variety of natural options, varied doses, and an assortment of regimens. After countless hours, months, and even years of experimentation, I found the best natural medicines to alleviate the pain that plagued me. I still get pain when I overdo certain things that aggravate the spinal cord nerve endings or the area where I broke my back, but I am now armed with knowledge and natural remedies to mitigate the pain that once ruled my life. I also have a rewarding career as an author and manage a stunning Victorian-era orchard on my acreage. Although my time was once spent in agony and darkness, my life is now filled with joy and light.

I am happy to share with you the culmination of my more than twenty-five years of research, personal experimentation, and clinical experience in this book. *Pain Erasers: The Complete Natural Medicine Guide to Safe, Drug-Free Relief* showcases the proven natural pain erasers backed by science and personal experience, rather than theory, ad copy, or complex bodywork regimes. It is my hope and belief that the information contained within these pages, along with the correct use of the remedies I share, will transform your life as it has mine.

In *Pain Erasers*:

- You'll find simple ways to free your life from pain and determine which remedies will work best for you.
- You'll learn the best essential oils, herbs, nutrients, and other natural remedies for joint pain, nerve pain, soft tissue pain, muscle pain, headaches, migraines, arthritis, fibromyalgia, neuralgia, and many other types of pain disorders.
- You'll discover the exciting research that shows just how effective these natural painkillers can be.

- You'll learn the best way to take each remedy to yield results. No medicine works if it is not properly taken, yet that is exactly what most people do when it comes to natural remedies. They take them in the incorrect form, at an insufficient dosage, and too infrequently to yield results. I will teach you how to maximize each remedy's healing properties and share my pain protocols that get great results. I should know: they've worked for me and the thousands of patients I've worked with over the years.

If you are among the nearly 70 million Americans who suffer from chronic pain (an estimated 50 million suffer from chronic pain and an additional 20 million suffer from high-impact chronic pain that severely restricts their lives),[1] I am confident that you'll find improvement or relief within these pages. Considering that many of these people also suffer from addictions to painkillers, the research on these natural options could not be more timely.

Let's face it: few people have the time to sift through the studies or follow complex bodywork programs and arduous therapies, particularly when they are suffering. While these programs and therapies may have merit, they are beyond the capacity of many people. With *Pain Erasers*, you will be privy to proven pain-busting natural remedies from which you can immediately and effectively benefit.

Something tells me you are already an expert on pain and how horrible it feels, and that you simply want trustworthy guidance toward relief. While I discuss pain briefly in the first chapter, "What You Don't Know About Pain May Be Hurting You," I have kept it short because the last thing you likely want to read about when you're suffering is the theory behind pain. Instead, we're jumping right into exploring the types of pain you may be experiencing to better help you pinpoint the best remedies to help you find relief.

In chapter 2, "Erase the 20 Most Common Pain Conditions," you'll discover twenty of the most common pain conditions and what's happening in the body in each of these conditions, along with my Natural Pain Prescription outlining the best remedies for each pain disorder. These conditions include back pain, carpal tunnel syndrome, diabetic neuropathy, eye pain (such as macular degeneration and glaucoma), fibromyalgia, migraines and headaches, plantar fasciitis, PMS and menstrual cramps, TMJ syndrome, tendonitis, trigeminal neuralgia, and whiplash.

In chapter 3, "Heal Your Gut—Heal Your Pain," you'll learn about the exciting and cutting-edge research on the importance of a healthy gut in alleviating chronic pain. A healthy, microbially balanced gut is perhaps the most overlooked factor in treating or managing pain, yet, surprisingly, I haven't seen it discussed in any other pain book. You'll learn the best remedies to heal your gut to set the foundation for great health and a pain-free body for life.

In chapters 4 through 24, you'll discover many of the best natural painkillers available and how to use them for optimal results. If you're like most people, you may have tried some of these remedies but may not have used them correctly, not through any fault of your own, but because this type of information is largely unavailable. It's not listed on product labels and is rarely mentioned in books or other publications. You'll find the research behind the remedies, from birch essential oil to willow bark. You'll learn about a powerful remedy from the Amazon rain forest that you may not have heard about. You'll also learn about the pros and cons of cannabis to help you decide whether it makes sense for you.

In chapter 25, you'll find many other supporting remedies that help alleviate pain and inflammation. While they are not the stars of the pain-erasing show, they play important supporting roles to help you get the best results possible. These remedies include astaxanthin, comfrey oil or ointment, glucosamine sulfate, methylsulfonylmethane (MSM), and others.

In chapter 26, "The Pain-Erasing Diet and Lifestyle," you'll learn the fundamental information to help you maximize the results you get from the remedies that follow in this book. You don't want to unknowingly thwart your best efforts and the best effects of the natural remedies presented by eating foods that worsen pain. In this chapter, you'll also discover research-based information about foods that help alleviate pain when eaten on a regular basis, along with advice about the importance of gentle exercise and emotional healing, since movement and the healthy release of pent-up emotions can improve pain.

It is my hope that this book will give you the sense of hope that Dr. Rob first gave me and that, later, I gleaned from my research and experimentation with essential oils, herbs, and other natural medicines. I encourage you to try the remedies I've suggested throughout these pages and to stick with them to get the results I know you can have. I hope that this book helps give you the quality of life, free from pain, that you so truly deserve.

What You Don't Know About Pain May Be Hurting You

We've all experienced pain at some point in our lives, and, sadly, most of us have experienced it on many occasions. From the first time we trip and fall while learning how to walk to occasions when we suffer much more serious injuries, accidents, illnesses, or other types of pain, the unfortunate reality is that we encounter different types and severities of pain during our lifetime.

If we're fortunate, we feel only mild or short-term pain, known as acute pain. But for many people, pain can become chronic, often destroying their quality of life and ability to perform daily tasks. For some people, pain can be excruciating, completely disabling them and causing severe emotional distress.

While people often deal with pain by popping an over-the-counter drug or applying a cream to the affected area, frequently these options don't work or work only minimally. Because pain is different for every person and has a wide range of expressions and descriptions, it can be difficult to treat. Worse than that, many pain drugs have serious, health-damaging side effects that can be undesirable. Some drugs can cause organ damage and can even be lethal.

While pain is a part of life, knowing what causes the pain we're experiencing, or better yet, how to deal with it in the least invasive and most effective way, is a set of skills we can all use. And I think most people would agree that knowing how to deal with pain in a way that is harmonious to the body, and free of serious or life-threatening side effects, is priceless.

PAIN IS NOT YOUR ENEMY

Pain is usually a symptom of underlying issues in the body and, while it doesn't feel like your friend, it is not the enemy most people think it is. Pain may actually be a messenger to draw your brain's attention toward an area of your body that needs attention and healing. Unpleasant at best and excruciating at worst, pain is a physical experience that indicates tissue damage. It's the body's attempt to prevent further damage and to heal the existing tissue damage.

We experience pain when a signal travels via nerves to the brain, where it is interpreted. For example, if we put our hand on a hot surface, the body sends a message through the nerves in the hand that travels up the arm, through the spinal cord, and to the brain, where the brain identifies the sensation and sends a signal back to the muscles in the hand to pull the hand away from the hot surface. The brain also sends a signal back to the hand, registering the burning sensation so the brain can rally its resources to help heal the burn. These signals happen at a lightning-fast rate, so we barely notice a moment between them.

The good news about this communication system and how quickly it works is that it can be manipulated to interrupt these pain signals so we can significantly reduce or halt our pain altogether. We can use natural remedies that affect the brain and its hormonal messengers to reduce inflammation, improve tissue healing, and, ultimately, alleviate pain.

WHAT CAUSES PAIN?

There are many different causes of pain, but the most common ones are linked to bone or joint damage that occurs through wear and tear, as well as to nerve damage and injuries that haven't healed properly or fully.[1] And, of course, there are many other varieties that involve tendons, ligaments, or the circulatory system.

While some pain is linked to a single cause, more often it has multiple causal factors. For example, back pain can be caused by poor posture; degenerative changes to the spine; incorrect lifting or carrying of heavy objects; being overweight (since additional weight adds extra pressure to the joints and bones); incorrect curvature of the spine; an injury from a sport, car accident, or other trauma; sleeping on a poor mattress or with insufficient pillow support for your neck; wearing high heels (see the "Reasons to Skip High Heels" box on page 12); experiencing severe or chronic stress; or some other lesser-known or unknown cause.

Of course, there are many underlying health conditions that can also cause pain, including cancer, fibromyalgia, gallbladder disease, human immunodeficiency virus (HIV), multiple sclerosis, osteoarthritis or rheumatoid arthritis, and ulcers.[2]

The source of pain may be obvious in some cases, but in others it can be quite enigmatic, leading doctors on a journey of medical discovery as they attempt to find the mysterious root cause. For many people, such a process and the lack of knowledge about the cause of the pain can be highly stressful, as the chronic pain condition continues to cause suffering. Uncertainty about the cause of the pain can make it difficult to effectively treat.

It's equally important to understand that the inflammation you experience is the body's way of coping with an injury, trauma, or infection, or addressing a damaged area that needs healing. It means that your body is sending out white blood cells to the problem spot to fight infection, oxygenated blood to repair damage, and other fluids to cushion damaged cells in an effort to protect the area from further damage. While this process is normal and indeed healthy, when it continues for a lengthy period of time or when it continues throughout the body at a low-grade level, it can become a problem. Any damaged areas can become vulnerable to further damage over time or may not properly heal, and you may be left with ongoing, chronic pain.

It may surprise you to learn that in many cases your gut health, or lack thereof, may be playing a role in causing or aggravating inflammation throughout your body or in isolated places that seem unrelated to the gut. Yet a growing body of scientific research shows that the traditional treatments for pain may have overlooked, or even worsened, a causal factor for pain: the microbial balance in the gut. See chapter 3, "Heal Your Gut—Heal Your Pain," for more information about the gut-inflammation connection and to learn how you can restore great gut health naturally.

Of course, whether or not you know the cause of your pain or inflammation, have been diagnosed with a pain disorder, or are still undergoing diagnostic tests to determine the cause of your pain, I encourage you to try the remedies suggested throughout *Pain Erasers*.

Reasons to Skip High Heels

If you're opting for sky-high stilettos or even midlevel pumps, you could unknowingly be harming your health and aggravating pain. That's because, according to Ottawa chiropractor and pain expert Dr. Robert Laquerre,[3] as well as scientific research, high heels may be the root cause of many different health conditions, including:

Fatigue: Heels over two inches can increase lower extremity muscular stress that constricts blood vessels and limits blood supply to muscles and the brain, causing a reduced flow of oxygen and a general sense of fatigue.

Knee pain: According to a Harvard study published in the *Lancet*, wearing heels around 2.7 inches or higher is linked to a 24 percent increase in knee strain and pain.[4]

Bunions: Bunions are deformations that tend to occur at the base of the big toe, causing the normally straight toe to become directed toward the smaller toes. High heels force the weight of the body onto the front of the foot, creating an increased pressure on the base of the big toe, which can make people more vulnerable to bunions. Bunions cause swelling, stress, redness, and pain.

Foot pain: In addition to bunions, Dr. Laquerre says that high heels are linked to numerous other foot problems, including metatarsalgia (pain in the ball of the foot) and Morton's neuroma (a thickening of the tissue around a nerve between the third and fourth toes).

Low back pain: "High heels force you to walk with the pelvis arched forward, causing hyperlordosis—a backward bend—of the lumbar spine," says Dr. Laquerre. This unnatural spinal curvature places excessive stress and strain on the lower back, which may result in lower back pain.

Nerve irritation: The unnatural curvature of the spine caused by high heels increases the pressure in the lower spine and can cause nerve irritation and reduce healthy nerve communication with the many organs and tissues these nerves feed. Since these nerves support the proper functioning of many organs and tissues, improper nerve communication or irritation can affect their ability to function in a healthy way.

Ankle pain: Wearing heels over two inches can create faulty biomechanics and place needless stress on your ankles, causing ankle pain or other ankle problems.

Hip pain: The same is true of the hips. High heels cause a forward pelvic tilt that can result in hip pain and strain.

Spinal problems: The unnatural curvature caused by wearing high heels can place a tremendous amount of stress on the spine, resulting in pain or spinal problems.

Types of Pain

There are many types of pain. Pain can be acute (short term) or chronic (long term); it can be local (in one part of the body) or widespread (in multiple places in the body). Pain is often described by the bodily part that is involved—such as joint, muscle, nerve, tendon, ligament, or bone—but it can also be described in terms of the conditions underlying it, which can include arthritis, cancer, multiple sclerosis, and so on.

Additionally, doctors usually classify pain by its level of origin: on the surface or just below the surface of the skin (somatic pain); from within the organs or cavities of the body (visceral pain); or perceived elsewhere in the body than the site of origin, such as pain down the arm caused by a heart attack (referred pain).[5]

It is helpful, wherever possible, to know the type of pain you're experiencing—acute or chronic, localized or widespread—and to know which body parts or organs are involved. This way, you can select the best pain remedies to yield the greatest results, rather than just pop them in an ad hoc manner, which tends to produce poor results. Before we explore the natural options, let's explore some of the problems with commonly used pain drugs.

THE PROBLEMS WITH PAIN DRUGS

Move over, Advil and Tylenol. Step aside, Aleve and OxyContin. If you take pain relief drugs, you may want to consider the effects of doing so.

Prescription drugs are the third leading cause of death in the United States and Europe.[6] The pharmaceuticals that millions of people turn to for relief from pain, inflammation, and other symptoms are not only causing side effects but actually damaging the health of many people. "Simple" nonsteroidal anti-inflammatory drugs (NSAIDs) are linked to a lengthy list of side effects, including bleeding gums, blood in the urine or stools, difficulty breathing, difficulty swallowing, dizziness, headaches, lightheadedness, and liver failure.[7]

Similarly, over-the-counter drugs that pain sufferers often pop like candy result in 30 percent of hospital admissions for adverse drug reactions, primarily due to bleeding, heart attack, stroke, and kidney damage.[8] Sadly, for many people, the problem is even worse than that. Every year, the side effects of long-term NSAID use cause 103,000 hospitalizations and 16,500 deaths.[9] Yet countless pain sufferers rely on these potentially life-threatening drugs to get through their days.

Prescription and over-the-counter medications also deplete your body of the vitamins and minerals required for basic functions. Over-the-counter pain relievers like aspirin, Advil, Aleve, Tylenol, and others on the market decrease your body's vitamin C, folic acid (vitamin B9), iron, and zinc. Steroid drugs like prednisone, hydrocortisone, dexameth-asone, beclomethasone, and triamcinolone are known to deplete pyridox-ine (vitamin B6), vitamin C, vitamin D, vitamin K, potassium, and zinc.

While that might not seem like a big deal, these deficiencies can worsen pain disorders by denying the body the building blocks it needs for tissue repair, which can indirectly affect pain. Additionally, these nutrients are needed to keep your immune system strong, maintain cel-lular integrity, build healthy blood and bones, heal wounds, and nourish joints, tendons, ligaments, and muscles. Without sufficient amounts of even a single nutrient, your body may struggle to heal injured areas and you may experience greater pain as a result.

Stronger prescription drugs, like opioids, which are usually pre-scribed for the most severe acute pain linked with major bone breaks or fractures, burns, cancer, and surgery,[10] are often associated with addic-tion and an extensive list of side effects. Some side effects of opioids are cognitive changes, constipation, delirium, itchy skin, nausea, and sedation.[11] You may have heard of some types of opioid drugs, including codeine, fentanyl, hydrocodone, methadone, morphine, oxycodone, and naloxone. When used incorrectly, in excess, or in "street" versions, they can be fatal.

Additionally, opioids, which are also sometimes called narcotics, can be dangerous when used in combination with alcohol, some antidepres-sants, some antibiotics, and sleeping pills.[12] Opioid use can also affect the progression of other health conditions, including chronic obstruc-tive pulmonary disease (COPD), dementia, kidney disease, liver dis-ease, and previous drug use disorder.[13]

Harsh prescription pain drugs can often leave people with worse health issues than those they intended to treat. Due to the addictive nature and potentially severe side effects of these drugs, most people find them undesirable.

While we could discuss the dangers of drugs indefinitely, and indeed there are many resources on this topic that I encourage you to read, this is not a book about drugs. It's a book about natural, safer options you can use in the treatment of your pain conditions.

Stress and the Emotional Effects of Pain

Stress can take its toll on any aspect of our health, so it will probably come as no surprise that stress often aggravates pain conditions.

In an article published by the Arthritis Foundation titled "The Emotion-Pain Connection," David Buxton, MD, shares his view that "chronic pain and emotions are so intertwined that it's often hard to tell where one ends and the other begins." Buxton states that "people with depression, for example, have about three times the risk of those without it of developing pain." Conversely, he adds, "those with chronic pain have about the same increase in risk for winding up with clinical depression."[14]

For those suffering from pain or depression, the situation can feel like a vicious cycle that is hard to break. It is important to remind yourself during these times that your view may be clouded by pain and that there are natural remedies and strategies that can help you cope with both the stress and pain.

It can feel like there isn't much that can be done about stress other than removing the source of the stress in our lives. However, there are actually many dietary and lifestyle strategies, as well as natural remedies, that can help our bodies cope with the effects of stress or reduce the amount of stress we're experiencing. You'll find lots of these strategies and remedies presented in chapter 26.

PAIN ERASERS CAN HELP

Whether you're suffering from acute or chronic pain; bone, joint, or nerve pain; or any other type of pain, the natural remedies presented throughout *Pain Erasers* can help. Of course, you should consult with your physician before changing or discontinuing your medication, add-ing new remedies, or altering your dietary, remedy, or exercise regimes. While *Pain Erasers* is meant to assist you in pain management, it is not intended as an alternative to a qualified health professional. Similarly, if you have pain that has not been diagnosed by a qualified health pro-fessional, it is important to do so to ensure you're focusing on the cor-rect condition and to rule out other conditions. Additionally, if you're dealing with opioid addiction, you should not attempt to discontinue opioids without qualified, professional guidance and supervision to help you address any withdrawal or other symptoms.

Rate Your Pain

Before starting any new pain remedy, including those listed in the fol-lowing chapters of this book, I encourage you to rate your pain on a scale of 0 to 10, with 0 representing no pain and 10 being the worst pain you've ever experienced. For example, if you suffer from excruciating migraines and you feel unimaginable, unspeakable pain, then rate them as a 10. Rate the pain that you normally experience at this time in your life, then rate your pain again one and two months later.

Write the pain rate number and date here: _____

_____

Write the pain rate number and date here (one month later): _____

_____

Write the pain rate number and date here (two months later): _____

_____

Feel free to keep a journal where you can rate your pain more frequently—on a weekly basis, for example, or even daily. Most people experience gradual improvements in their pain levels when they use the natural remedies showcased throughout *Pain Erasers*. There are multi-ple reasons to rate your pain. First, while some people experience sig-nificant and rapid pain relief, it can be difficult to observe the changes if they happen gradually. It's a bit like losing weight. Without a scale, most people wouldn't notice a pound or two lost, but the scale lets them know they've lost weight before the results become more noticeable. So rating your pain helps you observe the gradual changes.

Second, rating your pain and seeing the number drop over time gives you motivation to continue using the remedy or remedies you've selected, since you can better gauge their effectiveness.

Third, rating your pain levels and observing changes helps you fine-tune your pain relief regimen to get the results that work best for you. For example, if you rate your pain initially at a 10 and then at a 5 after only a few days of using copaiba (which you'll learn more about in chapter 9), you'll know it works for you and is best kept in your regimen. If you use MSM (one of the supporting remedies in chapter 25), which takes two to three months to produce observable changes since it works on healing the joints, a pain rating of 9 which reduces to a pain rating of 4 after a few months of use will indicate that it has been helpful. Let's face it: most of us can't recall the things we did only days earlier, so it is easy to forget the things we did a few months prior. Rating your pain level before starting remedies and then every week, or every month, as you use them can help you create the pain relief regimen that works best for you.

Using Natural Medicines for Healing

Most people have the misguided notion that natural remedies are not as effective as pharmaceutical drugs. Indeed, the multibillion-dollar pharmaceutical giants benefit from this myth. The reality is that there are many impressive natural painkillers that not only improve symptoms but also help the body heal the underlying causes of the pain. That's not the realm of drugs, which typically only work on the symptoms of pain or inflammation, or block pain signals between the brain and the body. Drugs are simply not designed for *healing* the body.

And while the general public is largely unaware of the healing potency of herbs and the essential oils and nutritional supplements extracted from them, the pharmaceutical industry knows how impressive they are. Scientists at various companies scour the earth for new plant compounds that they can extract, synthesize, patent, and then manufacture into so-called wonder drugs that promise to reverse or cure our worst health conditions. In reality, these pharmaceutical giants separate out a single compound from an herb and make a synthetic version in a laboratory, creating drugs with outrageous price tags and even more outrageous side effects. Some of these drugs are addictive, and some can even cause death, even when used as directed. As you learned earlier, the third leading cause of death in the United States and Europe is the *correct* use of drugs, killing hundreds of thousands of people every year. Imagine what happens when the drugs are *incorrectly* used—the problems magnify.

The process of singling out one compound found in an herb can also lessen the compound's effectiveness. That's because most herbs (and the essential oils and other remedies made from them) contain a hundred or more compounds that work synergistically to improve the effectiveness of the so-called active ingredient. While one compound often gets all the credit, there are usually many others working in the background to assist the absorption and utilization of the pain-alleviating compound.

I'm not suggesting that there is no place for pharmaceutical drugs, but complete reliance on this system is failing many people, leading them to suffer needlessly from side effects or become addicted to the substances they turned to for symptom relief. While the pharmaceutical-based system of medicine has a strong role in dealing with emergencies, it is important to understand its drawbacks as well.

Natural medicines, when used correctly, are far safer than drugs. Natural options have few side effects and, with some expert guidance, can provide pain relief as effectively as—or even *more* effectively than—drugs. And, unlike pharmaceutical drugs that frequently cost people their life savings, most natural medicines are affordable. They are usually readily available and don't require prescriptions. Most people will also be surprised to learn that there are effective natural options for nearly every condition from which they may be suffering. The growing body of research demonstrates their effectiveness even with conditions that are difficult to manage.

You deserve to live your life free of the pain that holds you back and causes needless suffering. Herbs, essential oils, and other natural remedies offer the hope and help you may need to alleviate your painful condition and start living life to its fullest. I have personally witnessed the restoration of health for people who make the effort to use natural remedies.

On the flip side, I've also seen many people who go to their local drugstore or department store, use a natural remedy a few times, and then report back that they tried it without relief. Some people even seem to wear the "I've tried everything and nothing worked" claim as a badge of honor, often relegating the natural option to the trash pile even before they've used it properly. Sometimes I've advised patients to use a specific remedy in a particular dose, three times daily, and to follow dietary and lifestyle recommendations, only to have them report back that my program didn't work. Upon review, I learned that they didn't actually take the full dose I recommended, may have substituted a cheaper (and less effective) brand of supplement, didn't take it every day, and gave up on it long before I asked them to. When they told me my program didn't work, I reminded them that the way they used the remedy was not part of my program and informed them that, actually, it was *their* program that didn't work. I encouraged them to try mine for the first time. When they followed the directions, using the high-quality products I suggested, they returned with much better results.

The reality is that even the greatest miracle medicines don't work when they are not used correctly, so it's important to find the high-quality products I've suggested in the following chapters, take them in the recommended dosages, and continue taking them as directed for the duration advised. Following these instructions, most people get rapid relief.

Many people don't get the relief they want from painful conditions because they use the wrong remedies. I can't tell you how many patients came to my office telling me that they used glucosamine sulfate for their neurological or muscular condition, but the remedy just doesn't work. No, it doesn't work well for these conditions, but it works well for joint health conditions, provided it is a therapeutic-grade product. This happens time and time again, with other remedies and other conditions.

As a result, I began compiling my personal and clinical experience with a wide variety of natural medicines, as well as reviewing the relevant research on them, and formulated a compilation of the best uses for the natural medicines. The reality is that not everything, drugs included, works for every pain condition. Some work better for nerve pain while others work better for soft tissue damage or joint injuries. You'll find this type of information for each of the natural options outlined in the following chapters. You'll also find detailed instructions on how to use each remedy to yield the best results.

I realize that exploring the realms of herbs, essential oil, and nutritional medicines can be daunting. That is why I've compiled my knowledge, experience, and research about the best ones for pain relief into a single guide to help you get the best results with the minimum amount of effort.

How to Safely and Effectively Use Natural Medicines

While most natural remedies are highly effective and safe, I will share some essential information to maximize their effectiveness and safety.

It is important to choose only high-quality herbs and essential oils, as lower-quality, inexpensive options typically have greatly diminished therapeutic effects. Worse than that, they may contain harmful ingredients that thwart your best efforts to reduce your pain. Sadly, most of the herbal and essential oil products found in department stores, drugstores, or bath and body product shops are low-grade, cut with cheap and synthetic ingredients, or contain toxic substances that are best avoided. Since you won't find these ingredients listed on the label, it can be hard to know if you're getting a high-quality product. Many herbal and essential oil products don't contain the effective species of plant.

This is especially true of essential oils in the marketplace, most of which are contaminated with solvents during extraction of the oil from the plant matter. Some contain inflammation-causing petrochemical products that are best avoided. Others have been diluted with cheap, unwanted oils that are not suitable for therapeutic use, particularly when they are to be ingested.

You'll also want to avoid products that are labeled "fragrance" oils, "perfume" oils, or "natural identical" oils. They are usually made from synthetic chemicals that offer no therapeutic value whatsoever. When it comes to herbs, essential oils, and nutritional supplements, you usually get what you pay for. For example, you could be thinking you're buying birch essential oil, but you may actually be getting wintergreen essential oil, which is much cheaper. If a product is cheap, it probably won't work and may actually aggravate your pain condition.

Where can you find high-quality herbs, nutrients, and undiluted essential oils? Keep in mind that while some companies claim their products are "pure" or "natural," there are no regulatory quality control standards that companies need to meet to make these claims. The essential oil market, in particular, is a bit of a Wild West when it comes to the large number of untrustworthy companies and potentially adulterated products. Purchase your oils from a company that specializes in essential oils and oil-related products and provides customers with extensive educational materials, customer support, and third-party testing of its products. I like and use dōTERRA essential oils for this reason.

Of course, as with anything, you shouldn't use herbs, nutrients, or oils that have expired beyond their best-before date as they lose potency over time and may have gone rancid. Choose a product that specifies the correct species of plant (which I've identified in the following chapters) on the label, keeping in mind that you may want to conduct some research to see if third-party laboratory tests confirm that you're actually getting what the label says.

While it is good to choose organic products, the reality is that the term *organic* means different things in the different countries where the herbs, flowers, or trees are grown, so it may not mean anything. Be sure that the herbs, nutrients, and oils you select are also sustainably harvested or manufactured to ensure that no environmental harm occurs in the harvesting or production. It may be difficult to discern how environmentally conscious a company may be; however, some companies, such as dōTERRA, are transparent in their materials sourcing and processing methods to ensure that they are meeting sustainability targets.

To ensure the potency, purity, and safety of your herbs, nutrients, and essential oils, store them in a dark place away from air, heat, and light, and of course, keep them away from children.

If you are pregnant or lactating, you should use only products that can be safely used during these times; most products have had insufficient safety testing for such uses and are best avoided.

Always inform your physician and obtain his or her approval for using any herbs, essential oils, or nutritional supplements prior to starting a regimen to ensure they are suitable for you, particularly if you have any health conditions, are pregnant, or are breastfeeding. Also, discuss any possible drug-remedy interactions with your doctor.

Don't discontinue any prescription medications without first consulting your doctor. And remember that herbs, essential oils, and nutritional supplements, while highly effective, should not replace any drugs you're taking.

The information and dosage guidelines provided throughout this book are intended for adults only. Do not use with babies or children without consulting a qualified health practitioner versed in natural medicine.

How to Use Essential Oils

Essential oils are highly concentrated and powerful natural medicines. By some estimates, they are between forty and sixty times stronger than the herbs from which they are derived, which means there are some unique safety considerations. A little goes a long way, so you'll need only a drop or a few drops at a time, based on the oil and the recipes I've provided.

It is best to use essential oils as directed on the product label or within this book. In addition to the safety measures presented above and with each remedy throughout this book, here are some other important considerations:

- Always dilute strong oils like clove, oregano, and thyme, among others, by using a carrier oil, such as fractionated coconut oil (a liquid version of coconut oil) or apricot kernel oil. A carrier oil is a gentle oil used to dilute essential oils to make them suitable for topical use.
- Conduct a skin patch test before using essential oils by applying a small amount of a diluted essential oil on the inside of your

arm and waiting forty-eight hours to determine whether you might have a sensitivity to the oil that presents itself in the form of a rash or hives. If you do, avoid using that oil either topically or internally as you may have a sensitivity or allergy to it. If you don't have a reaction, feel free to use the remedy as directed throughout this book.

- If you're planning to use essential oils internally, choose only products whose labels indicate their suitability for internal use.
- Avoid applying essential oils directly to the delicate mucous membranes of the eyes and mouth.
- When used topically, some oils can cause photosensitivity—that means that they can make your skin more sensitive to the sun. These oils typically include citrus and bergamot oils, which are not included among pain remedies; however, celery essential oil can also cause photosensitivity. Avoid using these oils on your skin within several hours of direct sun exposure.

There are three main ways to use essential oils: aromatically (inhaling their lovely scents), topically (applying them on your skin), or internally (either placing them on your tongue or consuming them in food, beverages, or empty capsules). Not all oils are suitable for all types of uses, so be sure to read the labels on the products you select.

AROMATIC USES

When you smell essential oils, you're actually breathing in potent oil-based plant extracts of essential oils wafting in the air. This sends signals directly from the cells in the nose to the brain. The brain then sends messages back to the body in response to the signals it received. These signals vary, depending on the scent (or scents) and its chemical constituents, and produce different effects—they can reduce inflammation, relax the nervous system, boost mood, reduce pain, or perform other actions. Inhaling essential oils is a quick way to allow their molecules to access the brain—usually in a minute or less. While this method is a powerful way to relax the nervous system, alleviate stress, boost mood, and improve sleep, it is less effective in alleviating pain than topical or internal use. That doesn't mean it isn't beneficial for use with pain conditions, but it plays more of a supporting role than the lead role.

The most common way to use essential oils aromatically is to place one to five drops in an aromatherapy diffuser. I don't recommend using oil burners as the heat can damage the chemical makeup of the oils, reducing their effectiveness and even causing them to smoke, contributing to health problems.

TOPICAL USES

Applying essential oils on the skin allows them not only to address localized or widespread pain conditions but also to quickly penetrate the skin and gain access to the bloodstream. Here are some of the ways in which you can use essential oils topically:

- Add a few drops of the selected essential oil or oils to a teaspoon of carrier oil like fractionated coconut oil. The level of dilution will depend on the oil and the skin sensitivity of the person on whom it will be applied. Apply the diluted oils to the affected, painful areas; avoid the skin around the eyes (unless you're using a product specifically formulated for this purpose), the eyes, the inner ears, and broken or damaged skin.
- Add a few drops of essential oils to a teaspoon of carrier oil and add to a hot bath. Soak for ten to twenty minutes to help alleviate muscle pain. Some oils that have strong heating or cooling effects, such as birch, clove, ginger, oregano, peppermint, thyme, and wintergreen, are not suitable for this purpose as they can irritate sensitive areas of the body.
- Add a couple of drops to an old face cloth that has been soaked in either hot or cold water and wrung out. Use as a hot or cold compress over painful areas. Cover the compress with a dry cloth to help retain its temperature. Do not use hot compresses on inflamed areas.

INTERNAL USES

Many essential oil practitioners lack an adequate understanding of essential oils as natural medicines, which often means that they discourage people from using one of the most effective means of pain relief—ingestion of suitable essential oils. I've used these methods in my practice for many years to help women and men put a stop to their suffering with exceptional results, even when little else worked. While some oils are not suitable for this purpose and there are safety precautions to consider, most people ingest some amount of essential oil in the plant-based foods and herbs they eat every day.

When done correctly, ingesting essential oils can be the most effective way to experience their benefits. Once you ingest a suitable essential oil, the oil compounds enter the bloodstream through the gastrointestinal tract, where they are transported to all the tissues and the brain to relax the nervous system, reduce inflammation, and quell pain.

As with anything that is consumed, it is imperative to use appropriate doses to avoid toxicity—the point at which even the healthiest of substances becomes unhealthy or harmful. If you're considering using essential oils internally, you'll need to determine whether the oils are suitable for internal use and, if so, how much to use and in which format—whether it is a capsule or a drop of oil taken directly or under the tongue, or another method.

Finding the highest-quality essential oils is even more important when you'll be using them internally. If the products you've selected are appropriate for internal use, they will have "for internal use," "dosage amount," or something similar on the labels. If the labels do not indicate anything like that, avoid using the products internally, since they are likely to have contaminants that are too toxic for such use.

Once you've selected the purest oils, you'll still want to check to be sure the individual oil is suitable for internal use. For example, some brands of high-quality peppermint are fine for internal use, but birch should not be used this way. I've included descriptions and information throughout this book to help you safely and effectively use essential oils. In the meantime, here are some ways to use essential oils internally:

- Place a few drops of essential oils in empty capsules, which are available in most health food stores. Take the capsules with a glass of water, along with some food. Some oils, like cinnamon, clove, oregano, and thyme, need to be diluted with a little fractionated coconut or olive oil before ingesting. Follow the package label for the specific oil you've selected.

- You can also purchase preformed essential oil supplements to target pain, address the sleep issues that often result from pain, or fulfill other purposes. Again, it is imperative to exclusively choose products that are high quality.

Regardless of why you're using essential oils internally, start slowly, using only a drop or two at a time, a few times daily. Do not exceed twenty drops in a twenty-four-hour period.

Erase the 20 Most Common
Pain Conditions

It's not enough to know about the best natural pain remedies. You need to know how to use them to get great results in your body. The reality is that nothing works well if it is not used in sufficient doses, with great enough frequency, for a long enough period. And with plant medicines, you also need to ensure you're getting the right species of plant, in the best format (tea, extract, decoction, essential oil, or supplement), and in the correct way (topically, internally, diffused, or via another method). In addition, you must consider whether the whole plant, an alcohol extract (also known as a tincture), an essential oil extract, or a standardized extract (a prepared product in which an active ingredient is added to a supplement to reach a certain percentage of the total product) would be the most effective way to use the remedy.

In this chapter, we'll explore many of the most common pain conditions and what's happening in the body in each of these conditions, along with a Natural Pain Prescription outlining the best remedies and the most suitable applications for each remedy and pain disorder, so you can put the most effective remedies to use in the best possible way to get the greatest results.

The remedies are divided into two sections: (1) Leading Remedies and (2) Supporting Remedies. While most internet, magazine, or newspaper articles cite many remedies as being great for almost any condition, the reality is that some remedies are better than others. For example, copaiba, which is largely unknown, may rank high for easing pain for those who use it, while MSM, which many more people take on a regular basis, is helpful for maintaining the health of joints but isn't necessarily the best anti-pain remedy. Similarly, consider that some remedies work marvelously for joint pain but aren't great for nerve pain.

I have divided the remedies into leading and supporting roles they can play for your specific condition so you'll have a better sense of where to focus your attention and budget to yield the best results. That doesn't mean there is no benefit from using the supporting remedies. Most are highly effective for healing and maintaining the health of the body. They merely take a backseat role in pain management, although they may be useful for overall bodily healing. If you are suffering from joint pain such as arthritis, for example, MSM would be great for ensuring that your joints do not further deteriorate and would be ideal in a long-term joint health program, while copaiba would work more quickly to reduce pain and inflammation to help you manage the pain you experience. Of course, you can't have relief from pain without factoring in your long-term tissue health, but the goal is to first get relief so you can start addressing your long-term healing afterward.

I based my classification of these remedies on more than twenty-five years of personal experience, as well as current research at the time of writing this book. Future research might change my categorization of the remedies. But if you're in pain, you can't wait forever for researchers to have a philosophical debate about the value of the remedies and for me to decide which category they best fit. You need results and you need them quickly. Accordingly, my goal for this chapter is that you will find practical and accessible protocols to help you be free of the pain that is causing your suffering so you can live a fuller life.

Here are the pain conditions we'll be discussing in this chapter, in alphabetical order:

Arthritis (osteoarthritis and rheumatoid arthritis)
Back pain
Bursitis and other joint pain
Carpal tunnel syndrome
Dental pain
Diabetic neuropathy and general neuropathy
Eye pain
Fibromyalgia
Gout
Migraines and headaches
Neck pain and whiplash
Plantar fasciitis
Premenstrual syndrome (PMS) and menstrual cramps
Sciatica
Shoulder pain
Temporomandibular joint (TMJ) syndrome (jaw pain)
Tendonitis
Trigeminal neuralgia

While there are countless pain conditions, I have selected some of the most common and, in the case of conditions like trigeminal neuralgia, some of the most painful ones. If you don't find your pain condition listed, it doesn't mean you cannot achieve results. Unlike pharmaceutical drugs that are typically designed to treat only one type of condition, natural remedies usually work on many different ones. So you would likely benefit from reviewing similar pain conditions and applying the protocols outlined below. To get the best results, consider whether your pain is of a joint, muscle, nerve, tendon, or other type. Choose a condition that has some similarities to your own. For example, if you have bursitis in your joints, check out the protocol under arthritis.

It's not necessary to take all the remedies listed under each pain condition. Most people find one to five remedies that are ideal for them. Obviously, selecting most, if not all, of the remedies from the Leading

Remedies section will likely yield superior results in getting your acute or chronic pain under control.

Directions for usage are found under each of the respective remedies. For example, if you suffer from arthritis, you'll find a wide range of suggested Leading Remedies, including birch essential oil, cannabis, and clove essential oil. To avoid redundancy and for ease of use, I've simply listed the remedies and provided some basic information on their primary uses for the conditions below—internal, topical, and so on. Of course, you should refer to the How to Use sections in chapters 4 through 24 for the particular remedies you have selected under your specific condition.

While cannabis is included as a possible effective remedy option under the relevant conditions below, be sure to consider any legal risks if it is illegal in your state or country. I'm writing *Pain Erasers* from Canada, where cannabis use has been legal for several years, but that may not be the case where you're reading this book. Because there are so many possible ways of reaping the benefits of cannabis and countless products on the market, use the recommended product or products as directed at your local medical dispensary. No single product works for everyone, so you may need to try a few different options—salves or ointments, edibles, or other formats—to see what works best for you and your specific condition.

ARTHRITIS (OSTEOARTHRITIS AND RHEUMATOID ARTHRITIS)

Arthritis is a rheumatic condition that causes pain and inflammation in the joints. Rheumatic diseases and conditions affect the musculoskeletal system and can include abnormalities of the immune system. The term *arthritis* has become so common that we often forget how serious the condition can be and how many people are affected. According to the Centers for Disease Control and Prevention (CDC), an estimated 54.4 million adults in the United States have been diagnosed with arthritis.[1]

While there are numerous forms of arthritis, the two most common forms are osteoarthritis, which is a joint disease, and rheumatoid arthritis, which damages the connective tissue and joints in the body and is considered an autoimmune disease. In autoimmune diseases the body's immune system mistakenly attacks healthy tissue, which can include the joints but is often widespread throughout the body. Other conditions like fibromyalgia and gout are also classified as types of arthritis. See pages 44 and 48, respectively, for information on these two pain conditions.

Osteoarthritis

By far the most common form of arthritis, osteoarthritis takes hold when cartilage (a fibrous, elastic connective tissue found in joints and other parts of the body) begins to deteriorate and wear down. There are many reasons why this can happen, but two of the most common are injuries and excessive body weight, which puts additional pressure on the joints and the ligaments that hold them in place.

Rheumatoid Arthritis

Rheumatoid arthritis is a painful condition of the joints that is actually a bodywide condition. It most commonly affects the hands but frequently occurs in multiple places at once, and can even affect the fingers, elbows, wrists, and knees, although not every person experiences the condition in all these joints. For some people the disease is more focused on the hands, while others may experience something more widespread. While it often starts in middle age and is often considered linked to aging, many younger people experience rheumatoid arthritis too. Though the symptoms are primarily felt in the joints, rheumatoid arthritis can affect tissue connecting bones and joints in many places in the body. It can also be caused or worsened by nutritional deficiencies and even pathogens, such as bacteria, yeast, and fungi.

The diagnosis of arthritis simply means inflammation of the joints, but it doesn't tell you what caused the joint inflammation. While drugs may reduce the pain in some people, I'm not aware of any pharmaceuticals that address the underlying causes of the condition. Worse than that, the drugs may be addictive and are replete with many serious side effects, including the possibility of death in extreme cases.

Natural Pain Prescription for Arthritis

There are many excellent natural medicine options for both osteoarthritis and rheumatoid arthritis. The following are the leading and supporting remedies.

Leading Remedies

Birch essential oil
Cannabis
Celery essential oil
Chili/cayenne
Clove essential oil
Copaiba essential oil
Devil's claw

Frankincense essential oil
Ginger essential oil
Licorice root
Oregano essential oil
Peppermint essential oil
Thyme essential oil
Turmeric essential oil

Supporting Remedies

Astaxanthin
Chondroitin sulfate
Comfrey oil, ointment, salve, or cream
Feverfew
Glucosamine sulfate
Guggul gum
Lavender essential oil

Marjoram essential oil
Methylsulfonylmethane (MSM)
Omega-3 fatty acids (from fish, flax, pumpkin seeds, walnuts, or a supplement with DHA and EPA)
Rosemary essential oil

From a holistic perspective, there are numerous factors to consider in treating arthritis, including addressing the low-grade inflammation that accompanies and may precede the disease and is often linked to poor dietary choices, a lack of gut health, and possible infections. Learn more about how diet contributes to inflammation and how to switch to an anti-inflammatory diet in chapter 26. Learn more about the gut-pain link and how preliminary studies suggest a bacterial infection known as *Prevotella copri* may be linked to arthritis in chapter 3.

BACK PAIN

How many people have uttered some back-pain-related curse when getting out of bed in the morning, or after helping a friend move, or upon rising from their desk after eight hours of work, or after performing as an all-star weekend quarterback with a bunch of middle-aged friends? Your back is involved in just about everything you do, and when your back suffers, your life suffers.

According to the Mayo Clinic, back pain is one of the most common reasons people visit their doctors or miss work, as well as a leading cause of disability worldwide.[2] The signs or symptoms of back pain include muscle aches; pain that radiates down the leg; pain that improves with reclining; pain that worsens with bending, lifting, standing, or walking; and shooting or stabbing pain.[3]

When it lasts for six or fewer weeks, back pain is considered acute and was likely caused by heavy lifting or an injury. If it lasts longer than that, it is considered chronic back pain and is most commonly linked to diseases like arthritis or osteoporosis, or to muscle or ligament strains, bulging or ruptured disks, or musculoskeletal irregularities.[4] If you suffer from arthritis, be sure to check out the section on arthritis on page 32.

Smoking, excess weight,[5] eating an inflammatory diet and insufficient amounts of nutrient-rich foods, a lack of physical activity or poor body mechanics during exercise, and other factors can exacerbate the condition. As a result, it's imperative to quit smoking, exercise regularly, build muscle strength and flexibility, and make an effort to maintain a healthy weight. Regular chiropractic adjustments or massage may be helpful in addressing musculoskeletal irregularities.

Natural Pain Prescription for Back Pain

There are many excellent natural medicine options for back pain. The following are the leading and supporting remedies. If you have arthritis in your back, follow the Natural Pain Prescription for arthritis found on page 34.

Leading Remedies

Birch essential oil

Cannabis

Chili/cayenne

Comfrey oil, ointment, salve, or cream

Copaiba essential oil

Devil's claw

Frankincense essential oil

Ginger essential oil

Oregano essential oil

Turmeric essential oil

Willow

Supporting Remedies

Astaxanthin

Chondroitin sulfate (if pain is linked to joints)

Glucosamine sulfate (if pain is linked to joints)

Methylsulfonylmethane (MSM)

Omega-3 fatty acids (from fish, flax, pumpkin seeds, walnuts, or a supplement with DHA and EPA)

Peppermint essential oil

Follow the dietary guidelines in chapter 26. And since inflammation is often the result of poor gut health, it is also important to address this potential factor. You'll find suggestions for doing so in chapter 3. Additionally, make a conscious effort to improve posture and body mechanics when you stand, sit, walk, or lift items.

If your back pain does not improve with rest, spreads down one or both legs, causes weakness or numbness in one or both legs, or is accompanied by unexplained weight loss, you should see your doctor.

BURSITIS AND OTHER JOINT PAIN

Bursitis is a painful inflammation of the bursae (pronounced bur-SEE)—the small, fluid-filled sacs that cushion the bones, muscles, and tendons. The elbows, hips, and shoulders, as well as other joints involved with extensive repetitive motion, are most often affected by bursitis.[6]

If your joint(s) feels swollen and inflamed, is uncomfortable when you move it or press on it, or feels achy or stiff, you may have bursitis. If the joint pain feels disabling or you are suddenly unable to move a joint, experience a sharp or shooting pain, have a fever, or experience excessive swelling, bruising, redness, or rash, then you should consult a physician.[7]

The most common causes of bursitis include repetitive motion or strenuous positions or movements, such as throwing a ball, lifting something over your head, or excessively leaning on your elbows or kneeling to perform tasks like scrubbing floors or laying carpet or flooring.[8]

Arthritis, gout, diabetes, or obesity can increase the risk of bursitis.[9] If you have arthritis or gout, be sure to check out the information and Natural Pain Prescriptions on pages 34 and 49.

Resting the affected joint to protect it from further damage is the key to healing. Bursitis will normally improve within a few weeks with proper rest. Of course, it is important to support the healing by eating healthy foods (see chapter 26), improving gut health (see chapter 3), and using some well-chosen natural remedies. Cannabis, copaiba, and turmeric are among the best options, although there are many effective remedies, which I've indicated in the following box. Additionally, make a conscious effort to improve posture and body mechanics when you stand, sit, walk, or lift items.

CARPAL TUNNEL SYNDROME

Having written twenty-four books and thousands of articles, I'm making an understatement when I say that I've subjected the nerves in my wrists to some repetitive strain. So it will probably come as no surprise that I have carpal tunnel syndrome, but I find that with some key

Natural Pain Prescription for Bursitis and Other Joint Pain

There are many excellent natural medicine options for bursitis and other joint pain. The following are the leading and supporting remedies.

Leading Remedies

Birch essential oil
Cannabis
Celery essential oil
Chili/cayenne
Clove essential oil
Copaiba essential oil
Devil's claw

Frankincense essential oil
Ginger essential oil
Licorice root
Oregano essential oil
Peppermint essential oil
Thyme essential oil
Turmeric essential oil

Supporting Remedies

Astaxanthin
Chondroitin sulfate
Comfrey oil, ointment, salve, or cream
Feverfew
Glucosamine sulfate
Guggul gum
Lavender essential oil

Marjoram essential oil
Methylsulfonylmethane (MSM)
Omega-3 fatty acids (from fish, flax, pumpkin seeds, walnuts, or a supplement with DHA and EPA)
Rosemary essential oil

essential oils, herbs, and nutrients, along with an anti-inflammatory diet like the one you'll discover in chapter 26, I can effectively manage the condition, enabling me to continue to do the many things I love, including writing books and blogs.

Known in the medical world as median nerve compression, carpal tunnel syndrome occurs when there is pressure on the median nerve that runs the length of the arm through a small tunnel (hence the name) in the wrist. This nerve controls all the feeling and movement in your hands, except the smallest finger. When there is excessive pressure on this nerve, the result can be numbness, tingling, weakness, and discomfort. People with carpal tunnel often find their hands and arms go "dead" at night, causing difficulty with movement and often intense pain, as well as countless sleepless nights, resulting in sleep deprivation. In severe instances, people may struggle to get out of bed. The condition can also result in difficulty holding things and periodic sharp pains in the hands.[10]

The condition is caused by repetitive movements like typing, sewing, knitting, baking, and hairstyling, as well as those involved in working a cash register or performing as a professional musician. Fractures and wrist dislocation injuries can also be causative factors. Carpal tunnel syndrome can be exacerbated by overuse or awkward wrist positions and movements, or an inflammatory diet, which is the type of diet eaten by most people. Women are three times more likely to suffer from carpal tunnel syndrome than men, probably due to their smaller wrist sizes and smaller carpal tunnels.[11]

There are many excellent remedies for carpal tunnel syndrome, which I've listed in the following Natural Pain Prescription. Some of these remedies are not normally considered specific for pain but can be highly effective for the natural treatment of carpal tunnel syndrome. A study published in the *International Journal of Immunopathology and Pharmacology* found that the herb echinacea combined with the nutrients alpha lipoic acid, conjugated linoleic acid (CLA), and quercetin effectively reduced pain and other symptoms and also improved function in people suffering from carpal tunnel syndrome.[12]

DENTAL PAIN

Dental pain, or toothache as it is more often called, is usually a sign of damage to the teeth. Tooth decay, cavities, a cracked tooth, or an infection in a tooth or gums can result in a constant dull ache, throbbing, or sharp, shooting pain. It can also cause tooth sensitivity that is aggravated by cold or hot foods or beverages, or sweets. Sometimes, it can

Natural Pain Prescription for Carpal Tunnel Syndrome

There are many excellent natural medicine options for carpal tunnel syndrome. The following are the leading and supporting remedies.

Leading Remedies

Birch essential oil
Cannabis
Celery essential oil
Chili/cayenne
Copaiba
Echinacea
Feverfew

Frankincense essential oil
Ginger essential oil
Lavender essential oil
Marjoram essential oil
Myrrh essential oil
Oregano essential oil
Turmeric essential oil

Supporting Remedies

Alpha lipoic acid
Cilantro essential oil
Conjugated linoleic acid

Quercetin
Rosemary essential oil

result in swelling and inflammation, redness, a fever, or a bad taste in the mouth.

Dental pain can be the result of fairly minor underlying problems or severe health issues, so it is best to consult a dentist to ascertain the root cause of your pain. Tooth decay is the most common cause of dental pain and is fairly simple to treat; however, it is wise to consult a professional to ensure there is nothing more serious going on. I've seen a person nearly die from septic shock due to a cracked tooth and the resulting infection, so it is a good idea to take dental pain seriously and get the necessary exam or X-rays to rule out any serious issues. Since tooth decay, fractures, and infections are all treatable, they should be the immediate approach in dealing with dental pain.

Tooth decay occurs when harmful bacteria damage the hard, exterior layer of the teeth, known as the enamel. The bacteria form a plaque that adheres to the teeth, making them more vulnerable to damage. Excessive sugar consumption can contribute to bacterial overgrowth that leaves your teeth vulnerable, so it is best to reduce the amount of sugar and sugary foods you eat or drink. That, of course, includes soda, which is one of the worst culprits for dental decay and bacterial overgrowth.

While there are many natural remedies that may be helpful for dental pain, clove essential oil is arguably the best one, particularly when it is diluted in a carrier oil and applied directly to the affected area. Refer to chapter 8 to learn more about how to use this remedy. Copaiba essential oil, diluted in a carrier oil, applied directly on the painful area can also be beneficial. Myrrh, oregano, and peppermint essential oils can be helpful to address any underlying bacterial infections that may be causing your dental pain. Add myrrh essential oil to your natural toothpaste. A drop or two of oregano essential oil diluted in a little carrier oil can be swished around in your mouth once or twice daily. A drop of peppermint essential oil can be directly ingested to help alleviate harmful bacteria and aid fresh breath.

Natural Pain Prescription for Dental Pain

There are many excellent natural medicine options for dental pain. The following are the leading remedies.

Leading Remedies

Clove essential oil   Oregano essential oil
Copaiba essential oil   Peppermint essential oil
Myrrh essential oil

DIABETIC NEUROPATHY AND GENERAL NEUROPATHY

Neuropathy, or peripheral neuropathy, is a condition in which the nerves outside of the brain or spinal cord cause weakness, numbness, or pain.[13] It typically occurs in the hands or feet but can affect other areas of the body as well. It can be the result of injuries, infections, exposure to toxins, inherited causes, or metabolic problems.[14]

Diabetes is one of the most common causes of neuropathy. Most people feel a stabbing, burning, or tingling sensation in the affected areas. Other symptoms vary depending on the nerves affected by the condition but may include gradual onset of numbness or tingling in the feet or hands; extreme sensitivity to touch; lack of coordination; muscle weakness; paralysis; heat intolerance; excessive or insufficient sweating; bladder, bowel, or digestive problems; and changes in blood pressure resulting in dizziness or light-headedness.[15] Neuropathy can affect

Natural Pain Prescription for Diabetic Neuropathy and General Neuropathy

There are many excellent natural medicine options for diabetic neuropathy and neuropathy. The following are the leading and supporting remedies.

Leading Remedies

Birch essential oil
Cannabis
Celery essential oil
Chili/cayenne
Copaiba
Echinacea
Feverfew
Frankincense essential oil

Ginger essential oil
Lavender essential oil
Licorice root (for diabetic
    neuropathy)
Marjoram essential oil
Myrrh essential oil
Oregano essential oil
Turmeric essential oil

Supporting Remedies

Alpha lipoic acid
Cilantro essential oil
Conjugated linoleic acid
Quercetin

Rosemary essential oil
Wintergreen essential
    oil

one nerve, two nerves, or multiple nerves. Carpal tunnel syndrome is
an example of neuropathy that affects one nerve. See carpal tunnel syndrome on page 37 for more information on neuropathy that specifically affects the medial nerve in the wrist(s).

Neuropathy is not just one condition; it is nerve damage that can be
caused by a wide range of conditions, including autoimmune diseases
(lupus, rheumatoid arthritis, Sjogren's syndrome, etc.); bone marrow
diseases (bone cancer, lymphoma, etc.); diabetes; genetic conditions
(Charcot-Marie-Tooth disease, etc.); infections (Epstein-Barr virus,
hepatitis B and C, HIV, etc.); and tumors.[16]

If you're suffering from diabetic neuropathy, work with a physician
when using licorice root, as the herb can also improve the body's use
of insulin and blood sugar levels, so you may need to monitor your
medication.

EYE PAIN

There are many possible conditions that can cause eye pain; some
of the most common ones include conjunctivitis (an infection better
known as pink eye); excessive wear of contact lenses and possible infections linked to doing so; corneal injuries (usually a scratch on the clear
surface that covers the eye); burns and toxic exposures (exposure to
chemical irritants or sun); blepharitis (infected oil glands on the eyelids); sty (a nodule formed by blepharitis infections); glaucoma (pressure inside the eye); optic neuritis (inflammation of the optic nerve,
which connects the eyeball to the brain); sinusitis (infection of the
sinuses); migraines (sharp pain in one eye can be linked to migraines);
and eye injuries.[17]

Eye pain can be serious, so it is important to seek medical attention
to determine the cause and to address any immediate treatment required.

Because there are so many possible conditions behind eye pain and
whole books could be written on each, I've selected some of the best
natural pain remedies. Keep in mind that these remedies are used internally or topically around the eye but not in the eye. See the section on
migraines and headaches on page 50 if you suspect that your eye pain
may be linked to migraines.

Regardless of the reason for your eye pain, the herb eyebright may be helpful in addressing immediate pain. Whether your eye pain is due to optic nerve damage, glaucoma, an infection, or something else, it is worth considering eyebright.

Unless you purchase a product that has been specifically formulated for use in the eyes, use the following remedies orally as directed in each relevant chapter.

Natural Pain Prescription for Eye Pain

There are many excellent natural medicine options for treating eye pain. The following are the leading and supporting remedies.

Leading Remedies

Alpha lipoic acid
Astaxanthin
Cannabis
Copaiba essential oil
Eyebright
Feverfew (if eye pain is linked to
   migraines)

Omega-3 fatty acids (from fish, flax, pumpkin seeds, walnuts, or a supplement with DHA and EPA)
Oregano essential oil

Supporting Remedies

Marjoram essential oil

FIBROMYALGIA

Many fibromyalgia sufferers live with chronic pain, fatigue, and other difficult symptoms that affect their ability to perform everyday tasks. Few have any clear indicator of the cause of their condition or, worse, how to address it or at least alleviate symptoms. If you're among the 6 to

12 million people, 90 percent of whom are women, suffering from the condition, you may be feeling frustrated with typical drug options, most of which have minimal effectiveness for this condition.[18] Fortunately, there are many effective natural approaches to the disorder.

Technically, fibromyalgia is a type of arthritis. Doctors classify it as a syndrome, which means that it is a collection of seemingly unconnected symptoms, with the main one being unaccountable pain in the muscles (*myo-* means "muscle" and *-algia* means "pain").

Here are the diagnostic criteria for fibromyalgia (however, you should get a diagnosis from your physician to rule out any other possible conditions):

- widespread pain in all four quadrants of the body lasting for at least three months
- tenderness in at least eleven of the eighteen specified tender points implicated in fibromyalgia
- generalized aches or stiffness of at least three anatomic sites for at least three months
- exclusion of other disorders that are known to cause similar symptoms

By definition, a syndrome is a collection of symptoms with an unknown cause. But we do know that fibromyalgia often starts after an illness, injury, or trauma. In addition to pain, there are often many other symptoms, including anxiety, depression, difficulty concentrating (sometimes referred to as "fibro fog"), difficulty sleeping, fatigue, headaches, itching or burning skin, lack of energy, memory problems, muscle cramps or twitches, and numbness or tingling in the hands or feet.[19]

Knowing so little about the syndrome, the medical community has had little to offer most fibromyalgia sufferers, but recent research could shed light on a major causal factor for the syndrome, which might help focus attention on what will improve symptoms. In a study published in the online scientific journal *PLOS One*, researchers found that insulin resistance may be behind fibromyalgia.[20] Insulin resistance is a reduced ability of the cells to respond to the action of insulin in transporting

Natural Pain Prescription for Fibromyalgia

There are many excellent natural medicine options for fibromyalgia. The following are the leading and supporting remedies.

Leading Remedies

Birch essential oil

Cannabis essential oil

Celery essential oil

Chili/cayenne

Clove essential oil

Copaiba essential oil

Ginger essential oil and herb

Marjoram essential oil

Turmeric essential oil and herb

Supporting Remedies

Bromelain

Frankincense essential oil

Methylsulfonylmethane (MSM)

Myrrh essential oil

sugar from the bloodstream into the muscles and tissues.[21] It is considered a precursor to diabetes and usually develops alongside weight gain or obesity. The scientists found that when they regulated blood sugar levels, they were also able to treat fibromyalgia-related pain, suggesting that the key to controlling symptoms, but perhaps also to managing the overall condition, is to regulate blood sugar levels and address insulin resistance.

Additionally, deficiencies in malic acid and magnesium are common among fibromyalgia sufferers. These nutrients support the muscular system and energy production at the cellular level and are essential for healthy muscles, so it is imperative to address a possible deficiency. There are many excellent nutritional formulations designed for the treatment of fibromyalgia that combine these nutrients. Ideally, select a product containing either magnesium citrate, magnesium malate, or magnesium L-threonate. You'll want to ensure a minimum amount of

150 milligrams of magnesium daily for at least two months for the best results, but most people benefit from 400 milligrams daily. Follow package directions for the product you choose.

Remember "an apple a day keeps the doctor away"? The adage may have applied to people suffering from fibromyalgia. That's because apples are a great source of malic acid and even reduce insulin resistance. Researchers at Tufts University found that the catechin polyphenols in apples contain catechins that improve the body's ability to use insulin.[22]

Effective Natural Remedies for Insulin Resistance

There are many excellent natural remedies to help improve the body's ability to use insulin, an underlying goal in the treatment of fibromyalgia, but cinnamon and ginger are among my preferred ones. You can add a spoonful of these spices to your daily cooking. You'll want to be persistent in eating them every day for at least a few months. They can be added to Moroccan-inspired dishes, Indian curries, or other foods, but I don't recommend sugary choices as the sugar will offset any benefits of eating these spices.

Depending on the severity of your symptoms and how long you may have suffered from insulin resistance, you may still need higher doses than what is available in dried or fresh spices. Both cinnamon and ginger can be taken in essential oil forms (be sure the products you select are suitable for internal use), which tend to be the most potent and concentrated versions of the spices, but due to their hot nature you'll want to add a drop or two of each to an empty capsule and take three times daily with food.

Cinnamon

Cinnamon has been used by herbalists for many years for the regulation of blood sugars and to deal with insulin resistance. Research published in the journal *Lipids in Health and Disease* found that cinnamon reduces high blood sugar levels and may help regulate other related symptoms.[23]

Ginger

Ginger can improve the body's response to insulin. Insulin is secreted by the pancreas to help regulate blood sugar levels. Research published in *Complementary Therapies in Medicine* found that ginger was effective in the treatment of insulin resistance.[24] Ginger essential oil is also a natural painkiller, making it doubly effective for the treatment of fibromyalgia.

GOUT

Gout is a form of arthritis characterized by severe inflammation and pain; it typically occurs in the big toe, but it can also affect other joints like the ankles, elbows, feet, fingers, and wrists. Those who experience it know that it can even make simple tasks like walking painful and difficult.

The condition develops when urate crystals accumulate in your joints; urate crystals, in turn, form when you have high levels of uric acid in your blood. The accumulation of inflammation and pain take the form of a gout attack. "So why is there so much uric acid in my blood?" you may be wondering. Your body produces uric acid to help break down foods that are high in compounds known as purines. Here are some purine-containing foods that aggravate gout:

- organ meats, such as liver and giblets
- red meat, such as beef, bison, and lamb; and pork
- fish and seafood, especially anchovies, herring, and mackerel, but also tuna, shrimp, lobster, and scallops
- poultry, such as chicken, turkey, and duck
- asparagus
- mushrooms

- alcohol, especially beer
- foods and drinks sweetened with high-fructose corn syrup or fruit sugar (fructose), including many soft drinks and sweetened juices

Under normal circumstances, when purines are eaten in small to moderate amounts, the uric acid dissolves in the blood and is detoxified by the kidneys; the uric acid is then eliminated from the body in urine.

Natural Pain Prescription for Gout

There are many excellent natural medicine options for gout. The following are the leading and supporting remedies.

Leading Remedies

Birch essential oil	Frankincense essential oil
Cannabis	Ginger essential oil
Celery essential oil	Licorice root
Chili/cayenne	Oregano essential oil
Clove essential oil	Peppermint essential oil
Copaiba essential oil	Thyme essential oil
Devil's claw	Turmeric essential oil

Supporting Remedies

Astaxanthin	Marjoram essential oil
Chondroitin sulfate	Methylsulfonylmethane (MSM)
Comfrey oil, ointment, salve, or cream	Omega-3 fatty acids (from fish, flax, pumpkin seeds, walnuts, or a supplement with DHA and EPA)
Feverfew	
Glucosamine sulfate	
Guggul gum	Rosemary essential oil
Lavender essential oil	

But if you eat too many purines or your kidneys are not functioning optimally, then uric acid can build up, causing urate crystals to accumulate in joints and resulting in pain and swelling.

Obesity is also a risk factor for gout, so losing weight can help you lower your risk of attacks. However, it is important to avoid extreme dietary programs since rapid weight loss can promote a gout attack. Additionally, it is imperative to avoid weight-loss diets high in animal protein, like ketogenic (keto) and Atkins diets, as they can aggravate gout.

While you'll definitely benefit from reducing the purine-containing foods in your diet or avoiding them altogether for a month to enable your kidneys and other detoxification organs to clear uric acid and start breaking down urate crystals, there are some foods you'll want to incorporate, including cherries and cherry juice; celery, celery seeds, and celery juice; and apple cider vinegar. Regarding the latter, be sure to choose an *un*pasteurized variety since it contains beneficial microbes that can help address the gut health that may be a causal factor in arthritic conditions. Apple cider vinegar also contains chlorogenic acid, which research shows reduces inflammation linked to gout.[25] Simply add a teaspoon to a glass of water and drink. Avoid using apple cider vinegar if you have an ulcer or gastroesophageal reflux disease (GERD). Additionally, while most of us know that we need to rehydrate daily, it is important for those suffering from gout to drink plenty of water to flush excess uric acid from the body.

Regardless of the number of remedies you select for the treatment of gout, I suggest using celery and copaiba essential oils both internally and topically on affected areas, according to the instructions outlined in chapters 6 and 9, respectively.

Be sure to see a physician if your inflamed and painful joints are accompanied by a fever, since this can indicate an infection.

MIGRAINES AND HEADACHES

If you've ever experienced migraines, you know how excruciating and debilitating they can be; anything that might help prevent them or reduce their frequency and severity is worth considering, particularly when the options are natural. And periodic or chronic headaches can make life much more difficult than it needs to be.

There are actually many types of headaches, of which migraines are one type characterized by visual disturbances, fatigue, disorientation, nausea, vomiting, pain in one side of the head, and sharp pain in one eye. There are two main types of migraines: common and classic. Both involve pain that is one-sided, is centered above or behind one eye, and usually begins at the back of the head and spreads to the entire side of the head; the pain is often accompanied by a stiff neck and tender scalp. They differ only in that common migraines do not include the visual disturbances, blind spots, light flashes, hallucinations, motor impairment, confusion, or difficulty in speaking or articulating words that can occur in classic migraines. Sometimes migraines are further

Natural Pain Prescription for Migraines and Headaches

There are many excellent natural medicine options for migraines and headaches. The following are the leading and supporting remedies.

Leading Remedies

Birch essential oil

Cannabis

Copaiba essential oil

Eyebright (as an adjunct treatment for headaches involving eyestrain or pain)

Feverfew

Peppermint essential oil

Supporting Remedies

Coenzyme Q10

Lavender essential oil (for stress, tension, and sleep)

Licorice root (if blood sugar issues are playing a role in migraines or headaches)

Magnesium

Marjoram essential oil (if headaches are accompanied with muscle tension)

Riboflavin (vitamin B2)

classified into other categories, including hemiplegic, basilar, retinal, and complicated. Hemiplegic migraines involve paralysis and altered sensations on one side, often accompanied by double vision. Basilar migraines usually involve slurred speech and complete or partial blindness. Retinal migraines involve blindness or blurring in one eye. Complicated migraines usually involve prolonged symptoms lasting a week or longer, or continuously.[26] Follow the instructions above for dealing with migraines. You may also find relief from chiropractic or craniosacral therapy if neck or head misalignments may be playing a role.

There are also many types of non-migraine headaches, including allergy/sensitivity, cluster, exertion, eyestrain, organic, rebound, sinus, TMJ/dental, tension, and trauma. The cause of most headaches is apparent in the name. For example, allergy/sensitivity headaches are usually caused by food or environmental allergies or sensitivities. For these headaches, it is best to seek allergy and sensitivity testing to find the root cause of your headaches. Skin prick tests, which are the most common types of tests for allergies, rarely discover food sensitivities. For the latter, some people report the effectiveness of a method used in alternative medicine known as Nambudripad's Allergy Elimination Techniques (NAET); however, keep in mind that this technique is still not recognized by mainstream medicine. Follow the remaining recommendations for migraines above.

Cluster headaches are sometimes called "suicide" headaches because of their severity. As in many migraine headaches, the pain is excruciating for sufferers. Cluster headaches predominantly affect men and involve agonizing, knife-like pain behind or near one eye. They are vascular in nature, meaning that they involve the dilation and constriction of the blood vessels. The pain is accompanied by tearing and reddening of the eye, drooping eyelids, facial flushing, sweating, and nasal congestion. Attacks tend to occur several times a day and may involve imbalances in neurotransmitter levels—hormones that regulate brain and nervous system communication. They tend to be worse in the spring and fall as there are changes in daylight hours. If you suffer from cluster headaches, it is imperative to reduce your alcohol consumption and cigarette smoking, avoid exposure to cold or hot winds, and, as discussed for allergy headaches, seek testing to find out which foods or environmental substances may trigger attacks.[27] For more information about balancing brain neurotransmitters, check out my book *Essential Oils for Hormone Bliss*. Follow the remaining recommendations for migraines above. You may also find relief from chiropractic or craniosacral therapy if neck or head misalignments may be playing a role.

Exertion headaches follow physical exertion such as heavy lifting, running, or sexual activity. They are vascular in nature, involving the constriction and dilation of blood vessels. It is believed that the pain is the result of physical exertion that induces swelling of the arteries and veins in the head and scalp, leading to headaches in people who are susceptible. Follow the remaining recommendations for migraines above.

Eyestrain headaches are obviously linked to eyestrain, so you'll want to reduce your exposure to computer screens and other technological devices, as well as fluorescent lights, and avoid long periods of focused visual work, such as artwork or reading.

Organic headaches are rare, experienced by only 1 to 2 percent of headache sufferers. They are the most serious type and should be ruled out by a physician if you suffer from headaches, as they can be linked to brain tumors, bleeds on the brain, glaucoma, swollen or diseased blood vessels, concussions, heart disease, or brain infections.

Rebound headaches, also known as holiday or weekend headaches, are linked to the rebound sensation when painkillers wear off or to caffeine withdrawal. Avoid overuse of narcotics. If you are reducing your use of narcotics, work with a physician to ensure you're getting the medical support you need. If you are reducing your caffeine consumption, wean yourself off slowly. Follow the remaining recommendations for migraines above.

Sinus headaches are caused by sinus infections and sinus pressure. Follow the instructions for eucalyptus (page 55) and peppermint (pages 159-162) essential oils as well as the remaining recommendations for migraines above.

TMJ/dental headaches involve facial pain that is primarily felt in the jaw and mouth, especially in front of and behind the ear. Consult your physician or dentist to determine whether corrective treatments are available. Apply copaiba and/or peppermint essential oils in front of and behind the ear and follow the remaining recommendations for migraines above. You may also find relief from chiropractic or craniosacral therapy.

All people experience tension headaches at some time in their lives. They are usually linked to muscle tension and stress. Follow the recommendations under "Natural Pain Prescription for Migraines and Headaches" to obtain relief and reduce their frequency.

Trauma headaches, also known as post-traumatic headaches, are usually associated with head injuries or whiplash. If you have experienced headaches that began after a car accident or other type of injury, consult your physician to address the cause of the headache. You may also find relief from chiropractic or craniosacral therapy.

The Surprising Cause of Your Headache and Migraine

Let's face it: most of us eat too much sugar. While sugar consumption is increasingly linked to a host of health problems, most people still don't realize just how harmful or addictive sugar is. While headaches and migraines often find their roots in other causal factors, sugar consumption may be worsening them.

Excessive sugar consumption causes rapid blood sugar fluctuations and the headaches that accompany them. Research published in the medical journal *Appetite* found higher levels of insulin in migraine sufferers.[28] Insulin is secreted by the pancreas, a long, thin organ that sits just under your lower left ribs, in response to the consumption of sugary foods. And, as most migraine or headache sufferers know, when your blood sugar levels drop due to lack of regular food consumption or about an hour after eating sugary foods, the stage is set for a migraine or headache to start or to become more severe.

Does that mean you should switch to Splenda or another synthetic sugar substitute? Absolutely not. Splenda (sucralose) has also been found to be a contributor to migraines in research published in *Headache: The Journal of Head and Face Pain*.[29] Stevia, a natural herbal sweetener, is the only sugar substitute that does not affect blood sugar levels.

Regardless of what type of headache or migraine you suffer from, there are some natural medicines that may be helpful, including cannabis, copaiba, and peppermint. If cannabis is legal in your state or country, use it as directed at a medical marijuana dispensary. Apply a couple of drops of undiluted copaiba essential oil to the back of your head, where your neck and head meet, as well as to your temples. (If you have sensitive skin, dilute the copaiba essential oil 1:1 in fractionated coconut oil or another carrier oil.) Apply undiluted peppermint essential oil to the same areas as well. See pages 107 and 159 for more information on use.

If stress or tension aggravates your headaches or migraines, also apply diluted marjoram essential oil to your neck and shoulders to help alleviate muscle tension that may be aggravating structural issues or putting pressure on the nerves and blood vessels to the head. See page 147 for more information on use.

If your headaches are linked to sinus congestion, sinusitis, or a cold that involves sinus pressure, you'll want to try eucalyptus essential oil since it works to clear the sinuses, thereby relieving the pressure that's causing the headache. It can be diluted (ten drops in a teaspoon of coconut oil) and applied to the chest. It can be applied neat (undiluted) to the palms of your hands repeatedly throughout the day and inhaled as necessary to ease sinus congestion. It can also be applied neat to a cloth that is kept on your pillow while you sleep to ease nighttime congestion. Use a cloth and a pillowcase that you're not concerned about getting oil stained.

It is imperative to make dietary adjustments such as those outlined in chapter 26 to address any type of migraine or headache. You should also manage your caffeine intake, as abrupt changes in caffeine ingestion can result in any type of headache or migraine. Try to drink your coffee or tea around the same time every day and try not to drink excessive amounts. While caffeine ingestion may temporarily improve a headache, when the caffeine wears off its absence can trigger a headache or migraine. It is a good idea to drink no more than three cups of coffee or black tea daily, but if you choose to reduce your caffeine intake, be sure to gradually reduce the amount you're getting; otherwise you'll risk triggering a headache or migraine.

No matter what type of migraine or headache you're suffering from, you may also be experiencing a magnesium deficiency, so it is important to supplement your diet with magnesium. This critical mineral is needed to ensure healthy communication between brain and nerve cells. Quite some time ago, scientists discovered that magnesium levels in the brain tend to be particularly low during a migraine attack, yet many doctors are not aware of this.[30] Additionally, scientists have known for years that magnesium levels tend to be low among women who suffer from menstrual migraines (migraines linked to menstruation); this information supports the use of magnesium in prevention and treatment.[31] While one study found that 300 milligrams daily improved migraines, most research shows that 600 milligrams daily are needed for at least two to three months for results. Keep in mind that with magnesium you're addressing underlying causal factors for migraines, not just providing immediate relief for pain that returns once the drug wears off, as in the case of most treatments.

Supplementation with coenzyme Q10 (CoQ10) may also be helpful for headache and migraine sufferers. In a study published in the *Journal of Headache and Pain*, researchers assessed the effects of three specific nutrients on migraines: CoQ10, riboflavin (vitamin B2), and magnesium.[32] The researchers found that this combination of nutrients not only reduced the frequency of the migraines but also significantly reduced the symptoms and their intensity. Study participants took 75 milligrams of CoQ10 in conjunction with 300 milligrams of magnesium and 200 milligrams of riboflavin.

Like magnesium, the herb feverfew also works best against migraines when taken regularly as a preventive measure, rather than for symptom relief. See page 125 for more information on how to benefit from feverfew.

Those suffering from allergy-related headaches, such as allergy/sensitivity headaches, cluster headaches, and migraines, may find allergy improvement from the herb butterbur. Known as *Petasites hybridus*, this traditional medicine is often beneficial for headache sufferers. Butterbur is available in most health food stores. Follow package directions for the product you select.

Whether you suffer from tension headaches or another form, stress and tension is likely a causal or aggravating factor. To help reduce stress and the muscle tension that accompanies it, try lavender, marjoram, and rose essential oils.

Highly effective at reducing tension and stress, as well as the headaches or migraines caused by stress, lavender is a great remedy choice. Lavender essential oil has been found in a study published in the medical journal *European Neurology* to be a safe and effective treatment for migraines.[33] Whether you're suffering from an occasional headache or debilitated by migraines, lavender, particularly combined with copaiba and peppermint, is a great choice. Rub lavender essential oil on your neck, head, and forehead. You can also diffuse it in an aromatherapy diffuser.

If your headaches are linked to stress and tension, diluted marjoram essential oil is an excellent choice to apply directly to the neck and shoulders, since tight muscles in these areas can often cause headaches. I find the combination of marjoram, copaiba, and peppermint particularly effective for this purpose.

Research published in the journal *Complementary Therapies in Medicine* found that rose essential oil applied to sore areas of the head and neck may be helpful in the treatment and management of migraine headaches.[34] It is an expensive oil but worth every penny as it offers profound healing, particularly when used alongside copaiba essential oil. If the rose essential oil you select is inexpensive, it is almost guaranteed to be diluted or cut with cheap or synthetic oils that are of no value. You really do get what you pay for when it comes to essential oils, especially rose oil.

Six Ways Diet Plays a Significant Role in Migraines

The old adage "you are what you eat" couldn't be truer than for migraine sufferers. Your diet may be playing a causal role or aggravating your migraines. Researchers at the University of Cincinnati College of Medicine pored over 180 studies to determine the role that diet plays in migraines.[35] They found that diet definitively affected migraines in the following ways.

First, the researchers found that monosodium glutamate (MSG) is a migraine headache trigger. MSG is found in many common foods, including soup (MSG is found in most soup bases and bouillon powder, even if the cook swears the soup is MSG-free), spice mixes, infant formula, baby food, soy "meat" products, bottled sauces and salad dressings, salad croutons, and protein powder, as well as in many vaccines.

Second, the researchers found that nitrites trigger migraine headaches. Nitrites are synthetic preservatives found in most processed meat products, including bacon, sausage, ham, and deli slices. Fortunately, avoiding nitrites is as easy as reading the label and avoiding foods that contain this additive. There are companies that make bacon, sausage, deli meats, and other meat products without this unnecessary ingredient, so it is easy to make the switch.

Researchers also found that caffeine withdrawal is a major factor in migraine headaches. Let's say you drink a cup of coffee first thing in the morning most days, but then the weekend comes along and you sleep in and don't get your coffee until noon. Your body goes into caffeine withdrawal, which often includes a full-blown migraine that will likely last the whole day but may last even longer than that. To avoid caffeine withdrawal migraines, try to keep the same schedule from one day to the next. If you are trying to cut back on caffeine, continue to drink a slightly lesser amount at the same time each day rather than cut it out altogether.

Researchers found that large amounts of caffeine trigger migraines. In their study, they found that over 400 milligrams of coffee triggered anxiety, depressive symptoms, and migraines. Each serving of coffee typically contains about 125 milligrams of caffeine, so limit yourself to three per day. Keep in mind that some brands of coffee can contain much more than that, so you'll want to check the amount in the type you drink.

The researchers also found that alcohol, especially red wine, is a trigger for migraines. While the researchers did not measure the difference between the effects of organic and nonorganic wines on migraines, the sad reality is that many vineyards growing grapes for nonorganic wines also tend to use chemical pesticides and fertilizers, as well as preservatives in their wines, all of which may play a role in causing or aggravating migraines.

The researchers also found that when omega-6 fatty acids were decreased in the diet in favor of increasing omega-3s, people experienced fewer migraines. Omega-6s are prevalent in safflower, canola, corn, and sunflower oils and foods made with them. Omega-3s are found in flaxseeds and flaxseed oil, walnuts and walnut oil, and hempseed oil. Learn more about omega-3 fatty acids on page 188.

NECK PAIN AND WHIPLASH

Most people have experienced neck pain at some point in their lives; however, just because you are in good company doesn't mean you have to needlessly suffer. There are many excellent natural remedies that can help. But first, let's explore the many possible causes of neck pain.

There are many bones (known as vertebrae), ligaments, and muscles that ensure your neck can support your head, move from side to side or up and down, and retain healthy mobility. However, muscle stiffness, poor posture, structural anomalies, injury, arthritis, fibromyalgia, or other factors can lead to neck pain.[36] See pages 32 and 44 for more information about arthritis and fibromyalgia. In rare instances, neck pain can be a sign of a heart attack or meningitis,[37] so it is important to consult your physician to rule out any serious issues.

Most neck pain is the result of muscle strain and tension due to stress, poor posture, long hours working at a desk without stretching or changing position, sleeping with your neck in an unsupported or awkward position, or jerking your neck during movement or exercise. There are many excellent stress management techniques that can help reduce the effects of stress, including deep breathing, meditation, massage therapy, sharing your experiences with a trustworthy friend or family member, and using essential oils like copaiba and lavender to help ease tension. Both of these essential oils can be applied to the affected areas, diffused in an aromatherapy diffuser, and even used internally. See pages 107 and 139 to learn more about how to use these oils.

To address muscle strain and tension, try to be conscious of holding yourself in a healthy, upright posture when seated or standing; take breaks from desk work or other types of work to stretch or change positions; get a good, supportive pillow that helps keep your neck in alignment; and be conscious of your positioning or sudden movements while exercising.

Structural anomalies such as scoliosis (curvature of the spinal cord) or an inverse neck curvature (an anomaly in which the neck vertebrae curve forward rather than forming the standard curve) can cause neck pain. These types of anomalies should be addressed by a qualified health professional, such as a chiropractor. However, many of the remedies recommended in this section may help with the pain and tightness linked with structural variations.

The neck is vulnerable to injury from car accidents, falls, and sports. The vertebrae can become fractured or broken, or the spinal cord can become damaged, all of which are serious injuries that need immediate medical attention.

One type of neck injury known as whiplash involves the forceful and rapid back-and-forth movement of the neck, like the cracking of a whip. It most commonly occurs in car accidents in which a vehicle is rear-ended but can also occur from physical abuse, falls, sports injuries, and other types of trauma. Most people heal within a few weeks of a whiplash injury, but some can suffer chronic neck pain. The symptoms of whiplash include neck pain; neck stiffness; aggravation of pain with movement; loss of range of motion in the neck; headaches (that normally start at the base of the skull); pain in the shoulders, upper back, or arms; tingling or numbness in the arms; fatigue; and dizziness.[38] If you suspect a whiplash injury, you should consult your physician.

There are many excellent natural remedies that can help with neck pain, whether it is linked to muscle stiffness, poor posture, or injury. Some of the best ones include copaiba, peppermint, and marjoram, but you'll find many others that can help in the following box.

Natural Pain Prescription for Neck Pain and Whiplash

There are many excellent natural medicine options for neck pain and whiplash injuries. The following are the leading and supporting remedies.

Leading Remedies

Birch essential oil
Cannabis
Chili/cayenne
Copaiba essential oil

Marjoram essential oil
Peppermint essential oil
Turmeric essential oil (for
   inflammation)

Supporting Remedies

Comfrey oil, ointment, salve, or
   cream
Devil's claw (if linked to joint
   pain)
Ginger essential oil

Lavender essential oil
Omega-3 fatty acids (from
   fish, flax, pumpkin seeds,
   walnuts, or a supplement
   with DHA and EPA)

PLANTAR FASCIITIS

If you're a runner, chances are you're no stranger to plantar fasciitis, a condition involving pain in the bottom of the heel. The plantar fascia is a thick, weblike ligament that connects the heel to the front of the foot; this band essentially acts as a shock absorber and support for the arch in your foot when you walk or run.[39] Plantar fasciitis can occur when there is too much pressure applied to the feet, resulting in inflammation or degeneration of this ligament. It is one of the most common orthopedic conditions.[40]

Natural Pain Prescription for Plantar Fasciitis

There are many excellent natural medicine options for plantar fasciitis. The following are the leading and supporting remedies.

Leading Remedies

Cannabis

Clove essential oil

Comfrey oil, ointment, salve, or cream

Copaiba essential oil

Frankincense essential oil

Lavender essential oil

Marjoram essential oil

Turmeric herb and essential oil

Supporting Remedies

Birch essential oil

Bromelain

Ginger essential oil

Methylsulfonylmethane (MSM)

Peppermint essential oil

Wintergreen essential oil

Plantar fasciitis involves dull, burning, sharp, or aching pain at the bottom of the heel or the midfoot region that tends to be worse in the morning or after sitting or lying down. The condition flares up during extensive activity, but most people don't feel the pain until after they stop.[41]

Plantar fasciitis is most common in runners and ballet and other dancers, but being overweight or obese and wearing shoes that don't provide adequate support are also risk factors. Of course, work that involves being on your feet, especially walking or standing on hard surfaces, can also put you at risk of the condition. Additionally, having high arches, flat feet, or tight Achilles tendons (the tendons that attach the calf muscles to your heels) can put you at risk of plantar fasciitis.[42]

Rest, ice, and braces or foot supports are usually recommended. In rare cases, your doctor may suggest surgery, but it is often avoidable with these treatments and natural anti-inflammatory remedies that support healing.

PREMENSTRUAL SYNDROME (PMS)
AND MENSTRUAL CRAMPS

According to a study in the journal *American Family Physician*, premenstrual syndrome (PMS) affects approximately 12 percent of women during their reproductive years.[43] I believe that number may actually be much higher since most women never report their symptoms to a doctor. Premenstrual syndrome, also known as premenstrual tension (PMT), can cause a wide range of symptoms, including breast tenderness; abdominal cramping and pain; anxiety; abdominal bloating; appetite changes; depression; and insomnia. While PMS is often the topic of jokes, the sad reality for many women is that it can be excruciatingly painful and even destructive to quality of life and the ability to work. When premenstrual syndrome is that severe and even debilitating, it is given the medical diagnosis of premenstrual dysphoric disorder (PMDD).

Whether you suffer from PMS or PMDD, you'll be happy to know that there are many excellent natural remedies that can help alleviate symptoms as well as address the underlying hormonal imbalances that are likely causing the condition. In my practice, women who declared that they had "tried everything" were astounded at how the correct application of these essential oils, taken in the ideal dose, transformed their lives.

Fennel essential oil warrants serious consideration for its research-proven ability to reduce the pain of premenstrual and menstrual cramping. See page 121 for more information.

Peppermint is an excellent natural analgesic remedy with widespread potential uses, including for neck pain, due to its natural constituents like menthol. It also contains a compound known as viridifloral, which helps restore estrogen levels in the body. Viridifloral is not specifically an anti-pain compound but seems to work instead to repair the hormonal imbalance that underlies PMS and PMDD.

In addition to the other remedies we've mentioned, clary sage essential oil warrants discussion. While not specifically an anti-pain remedy, this go-to treatment for female hormonal imbalances contains the compound known as sclareol, which, like viridifloral in peppermint, acts to regulate estrogen levels in the body. In other words, it addresses the underlying hormonal imbalances that may be causing your cramping and abdominal discomfort.

Essential oils combined with a low-sugar, reduced-meat, and more plant-based diet can alleviate symptoms (follow the anti-inflammatory diet outlined in chapter 26). Research published in the *American Journal of Epidemiology* from the Nurses' Health Study II at the University of Massachusetts Amherst found a correlation between diet and PMS.[44] The Nurses' Health Study II is a lengthy, wide-scale study that examines the effects of diet and lifestyle on health. The researchers studied the mineral intake of 3,025 women ages twenty-five to forty-two. Those women found to be eating a diet with the highest levels of iron from vegetarian sources (called nonheme iron) had the lowest levels of PMS at the end of the study term. Nonheme sources of iron include apricots, asparagus, bananas, beans, dark leafy greens, figs, kelp, lentils, peaches, prunes, raisins, and walnuts. Incidentally, most of these foods also contain vitamin C, which helps the body absorb iron. The study found that the risk of developing PMS was lowest among women who consumed more than 20 milligrams of iron daily, an amount that may require concerted effort to obtain from diet alone. Do not take an iron supplement unless your doctor has confirmed an iron deficiency. Follow package instructions for the product you select.

The researchers also found that higher levels of zinc may also play a role in PMS prevention. There are many excellent sources of zinc (you'll notice a lot of crossover with plant-based sources of iron). Some of the best food sources of zinc are beans/legumes, beets and beet greens, Brazil nuts (other nuts and nut butters are good sources too, but Brazils contain higher amounts), carrots, dark leafy green vegetables, onions, peas, pumpkin seeds, sprouts, sunflower seeds, and whole grains and breads made with them. Most adult women need about 8 milligrams of zinc; however, there really is no such thing as an average person. Additionally, your needs may fluctuate from one day to the next or during different periods of your life, depending on stress levels, whether you've been suffering from an infection, and other factors. Because both iron and zinc can be toxic in high doses, it is important to have your levels tested periodically if you're supplementing with these minerals.

Natural Pain Prescription for Premenstrual Syndrome (PMS) and Menstrual Cramps

There are many excellent natural medicine options for premenstrual syndrome and menstrual cramps. The following are the leading and supporting remedies.

Leading Remedies

Cannabis
Copaiba essential oil
Fennel essential oil

Supporting Remedies

Lavender essential oil
Marjoram essential oil
Omega-3 fatty acids (from fish, flax, pumpkin seeds, walnuts, or a supplement with DHA and EPA)
Turmeric essential oil

While low dietary iron and zinc are factors in the development of PMS, they are not the only ones. Vitamin B6 and essential fatty acids can often help reduce symptoms of PMS; however, it may take a month or two of increasing the amounts of these nutrients to observe changes in PMS symptoms. See page 188 to learn more about essential fatty acids that may help.

To learn more about balancing hormones linked to PMS, check out my book *Essential Oils for Hormone Bliss*.

SCIATICA

Sciatica is a condition in which pain radiates from the low back through the hips and buttocks and down the leg. It runs along the path of the sciatic nerve and typically affects one side of the body. Sciatica usually occurs when a spinal disk becomes herniated (compressed), a bone spur develops along the spine, or a narrowing of the spine compresses the nerves that run through the spine. It is characterized by inflammation, pain, and typically some numbness in the affected leg. The pain of sciatica can be severe; however, with treatment it often resolves within a few weeks.

In addition to the characteristic pain from the low back through the buttocks and down one leg, symptoms of sciatica can include tingling or muscle weakness in the same leg; sudden, severe pain in the low back; pain that follows a traumatic injury such as a car accident; and difficulty controlling the bladder or bowels.[45] The pain can range from aching to burning to a feeling like an electrical shock. In severe leg weakness or

Natural Pain Prescription for Sciatica

There are many excellent natural medicine options for sciatica. The following are the leading and supporting remedies.

Leading Remedies

Birch essential oil
Cannabis
Celery essential oil
Chili/cayenne
Copaiba
Echinacea
Feverfew
Frankincense essential oil

Ginger essential oil
Lavender essential oil
Licorice root (for diabetic neuropathy)
Marjoram essential oil
Myrrh essential oil
Oregano essential oil
Turmeric essential oil

Supporting Remedies

Alpha lipoic acid
Cilantro essential oil
Conjugated linoleic acid
Quercetin

Rosemary essential oil
Wintergreen essential oil

bowel or bladder changes, or following an accident, it is important to see a physician, who may recommend surgery.

Factors that can contribute to the condition include diabetes, obesity, and a sedentary lifestyle. Risk is also associated with occupations that involve heavy lifting, twisting, or driving for long periods of time.[46]

Regular exercise, maintaining proper posture, and using proper body mechanics when lifting objects or performing other tasks can be helpful in preventing sciatica and the pain involved with this condition.

Natural treatments include acupuncture, chiropractic, and massage therapy, to name a few. If choosing acupuncture, you'll likely get better results with an acupuncturist who practices Chinese acupuncture, rather than Western medical acupuncture, since the treatment for sciatica involves specialized Chinese needling, which is often extremely effective. Chiropractic treatments are also frequently effective, particularly for treating any compression in the spine that may be a causal factor. Therapeutic massage can also be helpful.

In addition, herbal and essential oil remedies can help address the pain and inflammation linked to sciatica.

SHOULDER PAIN

Anyone who has ever experienced shoulder pain knows how difficult it can be to perform basic functions. It can take a long time for shoulder injuries to heal because we tend to use our shoulders for many tasks.

The shoulder is a ball-and-socket joint with three bones: the upper arm bone, the collarbone, and the shoulder blade. Due to the unique arrangement of the bones, the shoulder has greater mobility than other joints in the body. Tendons connect the bones to the muscles, allowing for this extensive range of motion. The shoulder joints consist of four ligaments, cartilage, joint capsules, and bursae. The ends of bones are covered in cartilage to provide a smooth surface that cushions some shock. However, damage to the cartilage can make the joint more susceptible to wear. The joint capsule is a type of ligament that forms a bag around the joint to contain a lubricating fluid known as synovial fluid. This fluid helps keep joints lubricated. The joint capsule can be injured in the same way as other ligaments. Bursae are fluid-filled sacs positioned at key points around certain joints to act as cushions. They separate and pad neighboring tissues. High amounts of stress on a joint can cause the bursae to become inflamed, resulting in swelling. See page 37 for more information about bursitis.

Due to the complex nature of the shoulder and its joints, ligaments, and other parts, it is vulnerable to injury, damage, and inflammation. As a result, there are many possible causes for shoulder pain, including arthritis, torn cartilage, torn rotator cuff, swollen bursa sacs or tendons, bone spurs (bony projections that protrude on the edges of bones), pinched nerve in the neck or shoulder (see page 42 on neuropathy for more information about nerve-related pain), broken shoulder or arm bone, frozen shoulder, dislocated shoulder, overuse

Natural Pain Prescription for Shoulder Pain

There are many excellent natural medicine options for shoulder pain. The following are the leading and supporting remedies.

Leading Remedies

Birch essential oil
Cannabis
Chili/cayenne
Copaiba essential oil

Ginger essential oil
Myrrh essential oil
Turmeric essential oil

Supporting Remedies

Astaxanthin
Bromelain
Chondroitin sulfate
Comfrey oil, ointment, salve, or cream
Echinacea
Glucosamine sulfate
Guggul gum

Marjoram essential oil
Methylsulfonylmethane (MSM)
Omega-3 fatty acids (from fish, flax, pumpkin seeds, walnuts, or a supplement with DHA and EPA)
Rosemary essential oil

or repetitive strain injury, spinal cord injury, and heart attack.[47] The rotator cuff is made up of four tendons, which can become damaged or swollen, causing shoulder pain. Rotator cuff injuries involve the muscles and/or tendons that move the shoulder joint and give it stability. Because these muscles and tendons are involved in virtually all shoulder movements, they can easily be damaged. Tendonitis of the rotator cuff is the most common type of shoulder injury.[48] See the next section for more information on tendonitis.

Injuries can occur through sports, repetitive motion, manual labor, or excessive force. Shoulder pain can also be linked to spinal (neck) conditions, heart disease, or liver or gallbladder conditions.[49]

While most shoulder pain is related to injuries or inflammation of the various shoulder components, due to the potential seriousness of shoulder pain, it is advisable to seek medical help to discern the cause and treatment options for your condition, particularly if your shoulder pain is accompanied by chest tightness, dizziness, excessive sweating, pain in the jaw or neck, or trouble breathing.

The specific source of your pain or injury determines the best treatment plan, so it is best to get a diagnosis first. If you have arthritis or torn cartilage, see page 32 for more information on arthritis. If you have swollen bursae, see "Bursitis and Other Joint Pain" (page 37). If you have a pinched nerve, you'll likely benefit from chiropractic or massage treatments to help reduce the pinching. If the nerve-related pain is chronic, see "Diabetic Neuropathy and Neuropathy" (page 42). If your neck is the source of the pain, see "Neck Pain and Whiplash" (page 59). If you have tendonitis, see "Tendonitis" (below).

TENDONITIS

Many people experience tendonitis at some point in their life. It is the inflammation of the tendons, the tough bands of tissue that attach the muscles to the bones. Because tendons are not elastic, they're more susceptible than muscles to inflammation, especially from overuse. Tendonitis can occur anywhere in the body, but the most commonly affected areas include the hips, knees, shoulders, heels (Achilles tendons),

Natural Pain Prescription for Tendonitis

There are many excellent natural medicine options for tendonitis. The following are the leading and supporting remedies.

Leading Remedies

Cannabis

Clove essential oil

Comfrey oil, ointment, salve, or cream

Copaiba essential oil

Frankincense essential oil

Marjoram essential oil

Turmeric herb and essential oil

Supporting Remedies

Birch essential oil

Bromelain

Ginger essential oil

Methylsulfonylmethane (MSM)

Peppermint essential oil

Wintergreen essential oil

thumbs, and elbows. If you've ever experienced tennis or golf elbow, pitcher's or swimmer's shoulder, or jumper's knee, then you've experienced tendonitis.

Tendonitis is usually characterized by pain at the point where the tendon attaches to the bone. Symptoms can include a dull, aching pain when moving the affected joint or limb, tenderness, and mild swelling.

Tendonitis is often due to an injury that occurs as a result of overuse or misuse, so it is important to use proper posture and body mechanics, as well as to rest the injured tendons sufficiently to allow them to fully heal. The length of time you'll need to rest before returning to your activities depends on the extent and location of your tendonitis. When you return to exercise, jobs that involve repetitive motion or heavy lifting, or other activities that involve the affected tendon, be sure to start slowly.

Most cases of tendonitis heal with rest and natural anti-inflammatories and other natural pain-alleviating remedies (you'll find my preferred ones in the preceding box); however, in extreme cases, surgery may be warranted. If your tendonitis persists for more than a few weeks or months, it may develop into tendinosis, which can result in the deterioration of the tendon and abnormal blood vessel growth in the affected area, so it is best to see a physician if your tendonitis persists.

TRIGEMINAL NEURALGIA

Trigeminal neuralgia is among the most painful conditions a person can experience. It is a chronic pain condition that involves the trigeminal nerve, which carries physical feeling between the face and the brain. Even minor tasks like brushing your teeth or applying cosmetics can be enough to trigger excruciating pain for those who suffer from this condition. It usually begins with mild, short-lived attacks of pain, but the pain can increase over time. It usually affects women more than men and those over the age of fifty.

Symptoms can include shooting or knifing pain that sometimes feels like an electrical shock; spontaneous attacks of pain triggered by brushing teeth, chewing, speaking, touching the face, shaving, drinking, applying makeup, washing the face, experiencing a breeze, or smiling; severe pain in the side of the head or face that lasts several seconds or minutes; pain that lasts from a few seconds to a few minutes and usually affects only one side of the face; and an aching or burning feeling that sometimes occurs before the pain. The pain affects the cheek, jaw, face, lips, gums, and, to a lesser extent, the eyes and forehead.

Trigeminal neuralgia is caused by an impaired contact between a healthy blood vessel and the trigeminal nerve situated at the base of the brain. When the artery or vein applies pressure to the nerve, the pressure can cause the nerve to malfunction. The condition can arise due to aging, multiple sclerosis or another disease affecting the protective layer of the nerves (known as the myelin sheath), or, on rare occasions, a tumor. It can also occur due to a lesion on the brain, stroke, facial traumas, or surgical injuries.[50]

While trigeminal neuralgia can often be treated with anticonvulsant medications or Botox injections to reduce sensitivity to pain in the face, many natural remedies may also be helpful. Of course, if you experience severe facial pain that is not relieved by over-the-counter pain medications or natural pain remedies, you should see a physician. While serious causes of trigeminal neuralgia are rare, it is important to rule them out.

Just because the pain is typically agonizing for those who suffer from trigeminal neuralgia doesn't mean it needs to continue endlessly throughout life. There are excellent treatment options.

Natural Pain Prescription for Trigeminal Neuralgia

There are many excellent natural medicine options for trigeminal neuralgia. The following are the leading and supporting remedies.

Leading Remedies

Cannabis
Chili/cayenne
Copaiba essential oil
Eyebright (if the eye is affected)

Frankincense essential oil
Ginger essential oil
Myrrh essential oil
Turmeric essential oil

Supporting Remedies

Comfrey oil, ointment, salve, or
   cream
Lavender essential oil
Omega-3 fatty acids (from fish,
   flax, pumpkin seeds, walnuts,

or a supplement with DHA
   and EPA)
Rosemary essential oil
Willow bark

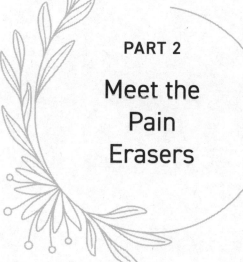

PART 2

Meet the Pain Erasers

Heal Your Gut—Heal Your Pain

N o current discussion on pain would be complete without a discussion
on gut health. That's because exciting research is beginning to show
that the gut may be a major factor in getting pain and inflammation
under control—even when the pain is localized somewhere else in the
body or spread throughout the body.

When you consider the pain in your elbow, knee, neck, head, eye,
or some other place in your body, you probably don't think about your
gastrointestinal (GI) tract. Unless your pain originates in your stomach
or intestines, you probably don't realize that your gut may actually be
implicated as a causal factor in your pain. Even pain that originated as
an accident or injury may be worsened by a microbial imbalance or an
unhealthy gut. A growing body of research links inflammation, which
is the root of most pain, to gut health, or to be more accurate, a lack of
gut health.

If you're like most people, you may assume that your elbow pain is
due to the overuse, injury, and inflammation in that area or that your

knee pain is linked to localized inflammation found in that joint. And while these assumptions may be true, they are likely not the whole story. You may not realize that the microbial condition and health of your gut is a significant factor in inflammation, and therefore pain, anywhere in your body, including that elbow or knee pain, or some other seemingly unrelated pain, and may play a role in whether your body can handle the regular use of the joint or if it will become weakened and inflamed. Addressing the health of your gut and any imbalances of microbes found there can significantly alter inflammation and pain elsewhere in the body. Before we discuss the ways to address microbial imbalances and ensure a healthy gut, let's first explore how the gut is involved in pain.

WHAT YOU DON'T KNOW ABOUT YOUR IMMUNE SYSTEM MAY BE HURTING YOU

The role of the gut is particularly important in pain disorders that are known as autoimmune diseases, or suspected to be autoimmune conditions. These are conditions in which the immune system wrongly attacks healthy tissue, causing pain and inflammation in the process. According to the American Autoimmune Related Diseases Association, there are over one hundred autoimmune conditions, including fibromyalgia, rheumatoid arthritis, inflammatory bowel disease (such as Crohn's disease or colitis), and endometriosis.[1]

Your body is actually a miraculous creation that orchestrates millions of biochemical and biological functions at any given time; heals wounds and broken bones on its own with almost no intervention from you; and grows new cells to replace old, worn-out ones every second of every day. So why would the immune system begin to attack itself? Sometimes, the immune system can go a bit haywire, overdoing its attempt to heal the body. Compounds known as inflammatory cytokines, or just cytokines, are released by cells to communicate with other cells as part of the body's attempt to heal infection or damaged joints, tissues, or other parts of the body. These hormone-like molecules not only encourage cellular communication but also signal the immune system to function when necessary and stimulate the movement of cells toward areas of inflammation in the body.

In the short term, cytokine production may help the healing process, but over time cytokines can become destructive to healthy cells. Cytokines may affect the cells from which they originated, affect nearby cells, or create a ripple effect throughout the whole body.[2] The malfunction of cytokines is involved in many painful inflammatory conditions and can become a vicious cycle. Cytokines can cause acute inflammation to aid the healing of a localized part of the body, but when the inflammation becomes chronic, inflammatory cytokines can wear down cartilage and bodily tissues, leading to further inflammation in the body, tendons, muscles, joints, or other type of damage.

In an effort to better understand the effects of cytokines, researchers conducted a study on healthy adults in which they induced the release of cytokines. They discovered that cytokines can cause anxiety, symptoms of depression, and cognitive disturbances. Cytokines also lower an important compound known as brain-derived neurotrophic factor (BDNF)—a protector of our nerve cells.[3] Getting cytokines under control is a key factor in restoring health and preventing or managing any painful inflammatory conditions.

HOW YOUR GUT MAY BE CAUSING OR AGGRAVATING YOUR PAIN

Since many inflammatory conditions start in the gut or are aggravated by conditions in the gut,[4] it is important to consider the health of your gut and to address any microbial imbalances or health issues that may be underlying your pain. While whole books can be written on gut health and the microbes that play a role in ensuring gut health, it's not necessary to become a microbiologist or gastroenterologist to start improving your gut health and to reap the rewards of doing so in the form of reduced pain and inflammation. This chapter is intended as an introduction to the topic, with some practical remedies and solutions for improving gut health. For those who would like more information about your gut and how to help it heal, check out my books *The Cultured Cook: Delicious Fermented Foods with Probiotics to Knock Out Inflammation, Boost Gut Health, Lose Weight, and Extend Your Life* and *The Probiotic Promise: Simple Steps to Heal Your Body from the Inside Out.*

The gut has a semipermeable lining, which allows the flow of nutri-ents into the bloodstream. Nutrients that have been extracted from the food you eat cross the lining of the intestines and go directly into the blood, through which they can travel to the locations in the body where they are needed for health and healing. Unfortunately, the gut can become excessively permeable, thereby allowing whole food particles, disease-causing bacteria, waste matter, or other inflammatory com-pounds to cross directly into the bloodstream, where they can wreak havoc, signaling the release of cytokines from the cells in the regions where these unwanted elements have traveled via the blood.

What Causes Gut Permeability?

Many factors affect the degree of permeability in the gut, including stress, a high-sugar diet or a diet with excessive amounts of animal pro-tein, and antibiotic or medication use, some of which are addressed by the recommendations in chapter 26.

Let's take a brief look at how stress can affect your gut health. Let's say, for example, that you've had a stressful argument. When you clash with your spouse, kids, boss, or someone else in your life, two triangular-shaped glands that sit atop your kidneys, known as the adrenal glands, pump out the stress hormone cortisol. These glands secrete cortisol in an effort to help you fight or flee from the stressful conditions.

While this mechanism is helpful in acute situations and may have been helpful in earlier times, allowing your ancient ancestors to run from a lion, bear, or other danger, the barrage of chronic stresses most people experience today causes the mechanism to overwork. Nowadays it's all too common to find ourselves in stressful situations: you experience stress when you stay up late to work or party, get news that your company may be downsized, discover that your spouse may be cheating on you, experi-ence the death of a loved one, or encounter any number of possible emo-tional or physical traumas. When stresses become chronic, the ongoing flood of cortisol can irritate tissue in the body, including the intestinal lining, which can become increasingly permeable when irritated.[5]

Additionally, any time beneficial bacteria are reduced or harm-ful bacteria or yeasts are increased in the gut as a result of stress;

antibiotics, birth control pills, or other medications; a high-sugar or high-protein diet; or many other factors, the stage can be set for the immune system to "sound the alarm." When this happens, the system increases the production of immune compounds like cytokines, resulting in further inflammation and intestinal permeability, or "leaky gut syndrome." The more permeable or "leaky" the gut is, the more toxins, incompletely digested food, harmful bacteria, viruses, and fungi have access to the bloodstream, where they may cause systemic damage and stimulate the immune system to attack what it believes are harmful invaders in the blood, potentially causing an autoimmune condition.

If the intestinal lining becomes repeatedly damaged due to ongoing or recurring leaky gut, tiny hairs that line the intestinal wall, known as microvilli, can become damaged and lose their ability to function properly. They become ineffective at processing and using nutrients we eat that are essential to digestion and our overall health. This inability to absorb nutrients can cause widespread nutrient deficiencies, which means that cells, tissues, glands, organs, organ systems, joints, bones, nerves, and so on can become impaired because the critical vitamins, minerals, and other nutrients that form the building blocks of these body parts are missing or insufficient. Without them, the tissues become weakened and more vulnerable to injury and may become inflamed.

Digestion becomes further impaired and you lose the ability to absorb other nutrients your body needs for tissue and organ repair and maintenance. You may become more susceptible to immune system attacks on the substances that permeate into the blood (the undigested food, toxins, etc.). Your body attacks these "foreign invaders" by responding with inflammation.[6]

It may not sound that serious, but over time this inflammatory response can lead to serious diseases as your immune system becomes overburdened and the inflammatory triggers continue almost constantly, damaging connective tissues, muscles, and other parts of your body, and thus initiating or aggravating pain conditions.

As an example, let's consider the health of your joints, which are linked to gut health. Osteoarthritis, for instance, has long been considered a joint wear-and-tear disease, but research is linking it to bacteria found in our microbiome. A person's microbiome is the sum of all the bacteria in his or her body. According to research published in the *Journal of Clinical Investigation*, poor gut health can lead to systemic inflammation, which can then lead to an increased risk of joint damage, as well as obesity.[7] And the obesity that is at least in part caused by an unhealthy microbiome means that increased body weight puts additional pressure on the joints, in turn aggravating joint conditions.

In another debilitating joint condition known as spondyloarthritis (SpA), researchers have identified a connection between intestinal inflammation and the disease. The scientists found that even subclinical gut inflammation is strongly associated with joint inflammation in this condition. While the research has not yet explored possible probiotic treatments of SpA, its connection to gut inflammation indicates the potential for probiotics to assist with the condition.

The Arthritis-Bacteria Correlation

It may surprise you to learn that research links harmful gut bacteria and the resulting gut inflammation to rheumatoid arthritis. Scientists at the New York University School of Medicine found an increased prevalence of the harmful intestinal bacteria *Prevotella copri* at the onset of rheumatoid arthritis. They believe these bacteria may set off an inflammatory response that begins in the gut—and may initiate rheumatoid arthritis.[8]

In their study, the researchers analyzed 144 stool samples from rheumatoid arthritis sufferers and healthy individuals who acted as the control group. They compared the gut bacteria of the two groups using DNA analysis and found that *P. copri* was more abundant in newly diagnosed rheumatoid arthritis patients than in healthy individuals or those with established rheumatoid arthritis.

The scientists also found that high levels of *P. copri* resulted in fewer beneficial gut bacteria in people suffering from rheumatoid arthritis, suggesting that both an infection with *P. copri* and a gut flora imbalance may be affecting people with the condition. While not specifically mentioned in the study, it is possible that the harmful infection was more capable of taking hold in the intestines of these individuals due to their lack of beneficial gut bacteria, since the latter work to keep infections at bay.[9]

If *P. copri* infections are linked to the onset of rheumatoid arthritis and to a lack of gut flora in the intestines, it is reasonable to assume that adding additional beneficial bacteria to expand their populations and diversity may help address *P. copri* infections. Whether or not it does, we know from many studies that probiotics demonstrate effectiveness in reducing inflammation by improving gut health.

While research into the effects of gut health on pain disorders is still in its infancy, most natural health practitioners have an informal saying: "Great health begins in the gut." We take the approach that a healthy gut underlies many of the body's ailments, pain and inflammation among them. This holistic approach is gaining traction in the research, so it's not surprising that many holistic health practitioners can attest that countless patients see improvement by taking this approach.

THE PROBIOTIC PRINCIPLE

The concept that inflammation begins in the gut in the form of a leaky gut, inflammatory cytokines, beneficial to harmful microbial ratio imbalances, insufficient beneficial microbes (diversity or population numbers), and harmful gut infections suggests a long-term healing strategy for treating pain and inflammation. It is unlikely to yield immediate or near immediate results for most people, but that doesn't mean it shouldn't be factored into a comprehensive pain management program. The results may mean less pain in the long term and a reduced chance of its return.

While there are numerous ways to heal gut infections, restore beneficial bacterial populations and diversity, and repair any gut damage, the process can start by taking a good probiotic supplement once or a few times a day and boosting the amount of fermented foods in your diet.

That's because the common denominator for inflammatory conditions is the fact that probiotics (beneficial microbes like bacteria and yeasts) in supplement form or the naturally occurring ones found in fermented foods are demonstrating their effectiveness for the prevention and treatment of inflammation.

To date, the research on the effectiveness of treating pain and inflammation conditions with probiotics has largely been done on gut disorders, immune system diseases, and, perhaps surprisingly, arthritis.

In one small study of rheumatoid arthritis sufferers published in the journal *Medical Science Monitor*, Canadian scientists assessed the joint function improvement in those who took the probiotic strains known as *Lactobacillus rhamnosus* and *L. reuteri* compared to those given placebos.[10] While the study participants taking the probiotics had significant joint function improvement, the researchers were unable to determine the mechanism behind the improvement. They concluded that the short duration of the study (three months) may not have been sufficient to identify the reason or reasons for the improved joint function.

Other animal research published in the *Journal of Interferon and Cytokine Research* found that supplementation with the two probiotic strains known as *Lactobacillus plantarum* and *L. salivarius* increased the body's own natural anti-inflammatories while helping to suppress arthritis.[11] *L. plantarum* is best known for its ability to reduce inflammation-causing compounds, making it beneficial in the treatment of diseases linked to inflammation, including arthritis. It is helpful in restoring healthy intestinal walls and is a warrior against some infections.[12] *L. salivarius* probiotics have been shown to have great immunomodulating effects,[13] which likely explains their beneficial effects for rheumatoid arthritis.

Exciting research published in the *Journal of Nutritional Science and Vitaminology* found that certain probiotic strains can restore balance to the immune system in cases of autoimmune disorders like rheumatoid arthritis.[14] The study found that a combination of five probiotic strains—*Bifidobacterium bifidum, Lactobacillus casei, L. acidophilus, L. reuteri*, and *Streptococcus thermophiles*—was more effective than other singular probiotics or three- or four-strain combinations.

Other research has explored the effective role of probiotics in the treatment of visceral pain, which you may recall is pain that originates from within the organs or cavities of the body. In a study published in the *Journal of Biomedical Science*, researchers found that the status of microbes in the gut dramatically affected pain levels and that altering the gut bacteria through the use of probiotics and prebiotics (naturally-occurring types of fiber and sugar that act as the food for probiotics, boosting the latter's effectiveness) could play a role in the treatment of this type of pain.[15]

While research into the gut-pain link needs expansion, waiting for the studies to pour in before you take action toward a healthier gut may not make sense. Most sufferers of chronic, severe pain would agree that they are not willing to wait to obtain the final stamp of approval on this gut-pain connection from the conservative medical community. And, considering that the effects of improving probiotic diversity and increasing overall probiotic populations in the gut have been found only to be highly beneficial, the approach warrants serious consideration.

WAYS TO BOOST YOUR GUT HEALTH

Improving gut health is the key to great health, regardless of whether you're dealing with pain and inflammation or some other health issue. The gut is so heavily involved in maintaining balance and health that it is frequently called "the second brain" by experts in the field. While poor gut health is common, in most cases it can be rectified.

Reducing sugar and artificial sweetener consumption also helps improve gut health. Sugar and artificial sweeteners have been linked to bacterial imbalances or yeast overgrowth in the intestines, which can lead to widespread inflammation. Reducing your consumption of these foods is a start toward greater gut health.

It's also important to eat less meat, as excessive meat consumption has been linked to the overgrowth of inflammatory bacterial strains in the gut, which can increase the risk of inflammation elsewhere in your body.

Add more fermented foods to your diet to boost your gut health, and add beneficial microbes that can help keep harmful ones in check. There

are many excellent choices, including yogurt or vegan yogurt, sauerkraut, kimchi, fermented pickles, and miso. Keep in mind that if the
product is sitting in a jar in the middle aisles of your grocery store, it has
probably been pasteurized and doesn't contain any live cultures at all.
Choose products whose labels say "live cultures" and that are found in
the refrigerator section of your health food or grocery store. And avoid
heating any of these foods, since most of the beneficial bacteria do not
survive high temperatures.

It's also a great idea to supplement with a probiotic that includes
strains like *Bifidobacterium bifidum*, *B. breve*, *Lactobacillus casei*, *L. acidophilus*, *L. plantarum*, *L. reuteri*, *L. rhamnosus*, *L. salivarius*, and *Streptococcus thermophiles*. While it may be difficult to find all of these strains
in a single product, choose one that has at least a few of these strains.

With a few dietary tweaks and some supplementation, it is possible to
have a healthy microbiome and improve pain and inflammation at the same
time. Refer to chapter 26 for more information and dietary suggestions.

To learn more about gut health and fermented foods, check out my
books *The Probiotic Promise: Simple Steps to Heal Your Body from the
Inside Out* and *The Cultured Cook: Delicious Fermented Foods with Probiotics to Knock Out Inflammation, Boost Gut Health, Lose Weight &
Extend Your Life*.

🌿

By now you have identified your type of pain (you know whether it is
acute or chronic, whether it is localized or widespread, and which body
parts or organs are involved); have learned about some of the most common pain conditions and found your Natural Pain Prescription; and
understand the importance of gut health and how it affects pain and
inflammation. Now let's bring on the stars of the show—the pain erasers. In the following chapters, you'll discover the best natural painkillers
available and how to use them for optimal results.

Birch Essential Oil

(*Betula alba, Betula lenta*)

We all recognize the stunning natural beauty of birch trees, with their white, paperlike bark and delicate leaves. The renowned Romantic poet Samuel Taylor Coleridge referred to this gorgeous tree as the "Lady of the Woods" for its beauty and elegance as it swayed in the wind.[1] Birch trees were viewed as the symbols of renewal, rebirth, and inception by the ancient druids.[2] But the trees are not merely the pretty faces of the forest. For many people they offer relief from pain and inflammation—and the potential for renewal.

Birch, like willow bark, which you'll learn more about in chapter 24, was used by Native Americans as medicine. Scientific research validated the use of birch and willow bark as natural analgesics, resulting in the latter becoming the basis of the drug aspirin, due to an anti-inflammatory and anti-pain compound, known as methyl salicylate, found in these trees and some herbs.[3]

In addition to methyl salicylate, birch also contains numerous other naturally occurring compounds known as betulene, betulinol, and betulinic acid,[4] all of which give birch essential oil its potent medicinal qualities. It is a powerful healer of painful joints and connective tissues, as well as broken or fractured bones, helping to rebuild these bodily parts while also alleviating pain in these areas.

Birch essential oil is used to treat rheumatoid arthritis and osteoarthritis, as well as gout.[5] It is also beneficial for sore muscles and general achiness, muscle spasms, and injuries.

Thanks to birch's active ingredient, betulin, the herb can also help with the mental stress and anxiety that often accompany either acute or chronic pain, as it works on receptor sites that help regulate one of the key neurotransmitters, gamma-aminobutyric acid (GABA).[6] GABA is a natural brain hormone that has calming and antianxiety effects, which can also help relax the nervous system.

HOW TO USE

Birch essential oil is best used topically on any type of joint injury or pain, including bursitis, gout, osteoarthritis, and rheumatoid arthritis.

SAFETY CONSIDERATIONS

Birch essential oil is not suitable for internal use. Avoid during pregnancy. Do not use if you suffer from epilepsy. If you are allergic to apples, celery, hazelnuts, mugwort, peanuts, soybeans, or wild carrot, you may be sensitive or allergic to birch, and in such cases, it is best avoided. While I don't recommend birch for internal use, you should also be aware that if you choose to use a birch product for internal uses, it may cause sodium retention, which can aggravate hypertension (high blood pressure).[7] Sadly, many "birch" products on the market are actually wintergreen essential oil, or a synthetic, laboratory-concocted version of wintergreen, which doesn't offer the same healing benefits of birch (and may offer no therapeutic benefits at all). Be sure to choose a reputable brand that provides third-party laboratory testing of the oil to confirm that you are, indeed, getting what you pay for.

SUPER HEALTH BONUS

Application of birch essential oil to areas with the type of sun damage known as actinic keratosis may help heal the affected areas.[8] Birch essential oil can also be applied to warts. Caused by the human papillomavirus (HPV), warts often respond to the antiviral compounds betulin and betulinic acid,[9] as well as salicylates.[10] Apply as directed above for either skin condition.

Cannabis

(*Cannabis sativa*)

Several years ago, the *New York Times* conducted a poll asking readers whether marijuana should be legalized. While I suspected that a lot of people favored legalizing marijuana, I was surprised to discover just how many. Out of 4,290 people polled, 41 said they were unsure, 206 were against legalizing marijuana, and a whopping 4,043 were in favor of legalizing the herb. Based on the results, journalist Juliet Lapidos stated, "The lopsided reaction indicates that, among *Times* readers, there's a virtual consensus: The federal ban on marijuana makes no sense."[1] And I can only imagine that today's results would be even more lopsided in favor of marijuana legalization.

In many ways current laws banning marijuana use are similar to the Prohibition laws in the last century that banned alcohol. And, with the clarity of time, most of us look back on those laws as being, well, rather backward. Some American states have legalized cannabis for medical use, and in Canada, where I live, it has been legal for a few years, which I fully support, considering cannabis's impressive track record of healing benefits, particularly for pain. While some people continue to debate the medical purpose of cannabis, it has far fewer health risks than most over-the-counter medications, which are, obviously, readily available. As a result, even the risk argument actually seems to favor legalization in the remaining states and countries where cannabis has not already been legalized.

Israel offers a great example of an effective medical cannabis treatment program. Nearly ten thousand patients with serious diseases and health conditions have low-cost access to up to 100 grams of the herb each month to aid their health.[2] The noncontroversial program is widely considered a success and offers a stark contrast to the high-priced pharmaceutical drugs in North America, where only the rich or those with excellent insurance plans can get access.

There are approximately five hundred naturally occurring compounds found in marijuana, or *Cannabis sativa*,[3] of which more than one hundred are collectively known as cannabinoids. Delta-9-tetrahydrocannabinol (THC) is the most well-known therapeutic cannabinoid and is the compound that is responsible for the high associated with cannabis use.[4] Cannabis also contains beta-caryophyllene (BCP) and cannabidiol (CBD), which are the compounds responsible for its pain-alleviating and anti-inflammatory effects. Neither BCP nor CBD has psychoactive properties. And while most other cannabinoids are unique to cannabis, BCP is also found in copaiba, which we'll discuss in greater detail in chapter 9, as well as in black pepper, cloves, hops, and rosemary in lesser amounts.

Recently scientists have found another compound in cannabis that offers analgesic effects. Called HU-444 by the researchers who discovered it, this novel compound demonstrated significant anti-inflammatory effects without the likelihood of the mind-altering effects commonly attributed to cannabis use. In a study published in the *Journal of Pharmacology and Experimental Therapeutics*, the authors state that "HU-444 represents a potential innovate treatment for rheumatoid arthritis and other inflammatory diseases."[5]

Regardless of the specific compounds at work, cannabis use has been found to alleviate the pain and inflammation in many conditions, including rheumatoid arthritis,[6] multiple sclerosis,[7] trigeminal neuralgia,[8] and even cancer.[9] It has also been so effective in the treatment of pain linked to glaucoma, which increases pressure inside the eyeball and can lead to vision loss, that some researchers are working on developing new drugs based on cannabis for treating the condition.[10] Natural cannabis products, in my opinion, are likely to be more effective and safer than synthetic, laboratory-derived drugs that barely reflect the plant's natural compounds.

Studies aside, I've had anecdotal reports of cannabis's effectiveness for treating a wide range of pain disorders, including diabetic neuropathy and other types of nerve pain, hip dysplasia, migraines, and sciatica, to name a few.

HOW TO USE

There are a wide variety of cannabis products on the market. Whole books could be written on the various products and the benefits and disadvantages of each. Smoking marijuana may be effective for some people and tends to have quick results, while ingesting oral options may, at least according to some research, have longer-lasting effects.[11]

While most people have reported to me greater pain relief from using THC products or whole cannabis products than from using CBD products alone, others prefer CBD products since they don't produce the high associated with marijuana use. This factor is particularly important if they need to use the product during their workdays or if they work in jobs that require abstinence from psychoactive substances. Applying THC balms, ointments, or salves directly to painful areas can also be helpful for people suffering from any type of pain (joint, muscle, soft tissue, nerve, or other). For this purpose, you'll want to compare the amount of THC in the products (ideally 200 milligrams for a 30-milliliter jar of ointment) you're considering or choose a whole-herb-based product. Use less than a pea-sized amount at first and wait two hours before reapplying.

It is best to start gradually and build up when using cannabis products, regardless of whether you choose to smoke marijuana, eat edibles, apply balms, or use some other form.

SAFETY CONSIDERATIONS

Cannabis is not legal everywhere, so you should be cognizant of the laws in your state or region. Obviously, cannabis is not suitable for everyone suffering from pain. Those with a history of addiction should avoid it. It can cause uncomfortable withdrawal symptoms in people who suddenly discontinue use.

Many people cite the potential harmful side effects of cannabis's long-term use as a rationale for keeping it illegal, but Canadian research on the matter might change their minds. In an article published in the *Journal of Pain*, scientists from the Research Institute of the McGill University Health Centre showcased the results of the world's first long-term study of marijuana use for pain treatment. The scientists dispensed a standardized cannabis product with 12.5 percent THC to 215 chronic pain sufferers who had not used cannabis prior to the study; 216 additional chronic pain sufferers who were not cannabis users acted as controls for the study. The researchers followed the study participants for one year to determine whether there was any potential for negative side effects of using the herb in the long term. While some members of the cannabis group experienced mild side effects after a year of use, there was no increased risk of serious adverse effects.[12]

There is a growing body of research about cannabis's potential for medicinal benefits, and this long-term research, which showcases its safe use with few negative side effects, suggests that marijuana's acceptance will likely continue its decades-long upward trend. Bearing in mind the potential side effects of pharmaceutical drugs for the treatment of pain, medical marijuana certainly warrants further consideration.

Avoid vaping cannabis, or using it in e-cigarettes, as this has been linked to a novel and serious respiratory condition known as e-cigarette or vaping product use–associated lung injury (EVALI), which can result in death.[13]

Use any cannabis product with caution or avoid altogether if you suffer from tachycardia (rapid heartbeat).[14]

If you experience anxiety, you may find cannabis helpful, as low doses have been found to improve anxiety; however, higher doses may aggravate the condition and may be linked to paranoia. And as anyone who's ever tried talking to someone who is high knows, memory impairment is common among cannabis users. Depending on the type of cannabis substance used, it may have mind-altering effects. This is particularly evident among people who haven't used it before, as well as many young people.

One study found an increased risk of heart attack within the first hour of smoking marijuana, so it is wise to consider this possible effect, particularly if you suffer from heart disease.[15]

According to scientists at UCLA, wild or "feral" cannabis tends to contain similar amounts of THC and CBD as commercially grown varieties, while cannabis seized by the US Drug Enforcement Agency over the last couple of decades has THC levels that may be ten to one hundred times greater than CBD levels. UCLA scientists suggest that this unnaturally elevated THC to CBD ratio may exacerbate potential health issues, particularly cognitive and psychiatric disorders.[16]

To ensure you're getting high-quality cannabis, it is advisable to obtain cannabis from a reputable medical cannabis dispensary with qualified professionals who can help you find the product(s) that are best for you based on your specific condition, work requirements, and other factors. I also recommend choosing the products with the fewest synthetic ingredients, artificial colors, and additives.

SUPER HEALTH BONUS

There are many potential health benefits of using medical cannabis, depending on your underlying health conditions. Marijuana may slow the progression of Alzheimer's disease, according to research conducted by the Scripps Research Institute and published in *Molecular Pharmaceutics*.[17] Research published in *MedPage Today* found that marijuana use eased tremors and improved fine motor skills in patients with Parkinson's disease.[18] Marijuana has been shown in research at Virginia Commonwealth University to stop seizures in animals, making it potentially helpful in the treatment of epilepsy.[19] A study published in the journal *Molecular Cancer Therapeutics* found that the cannabidiol in marijuana turns off a gene called Id-1, which cancer cells use to spread.[20]

Celery Essential Oil

(*Apium graveolens*)

The late botanist and author of *The Green Pharmacy*, James Duke, PhD, helped to make the anti-inflammatory properties of celery and celery seeds popular due to his recommendation for these foods in the treatment of gout.[1] In an animal study published in *Progress in Drug Research*, scientists found that an extract of celery seeds was at least as effective as aspirin, ibuprofen, and naproxen in the treatment of arthritis pain and inflammation.[2] And while celery juice gets all the publicity, there is a lesser-known but more effective way to reap the benefits of celery: celery essential oil.

Primarily extracted from the tiny seeds of the plant, celery essential oil is a potent anti-inflammatory that is particularly effective against pain conditions involving the joints, including both osteoarthritis and rheumatoid arthritis. Celery essential oil is also showing tremendous promise in the treatment of gout, a type of arthritis that involves the buildup of uric acid and is often felt in the big toe, making it painful for sufferers to walk. In an animal study published in the journal *Molecular*

Medicine Reports, researchers found that the ingestion of celery essential oil resulted in reduced uric acid in the blood, reduced joint-damaging free radicals, reduced joint swelling, and an increase in compounds in the body known as superoxide dismutase and glutathione.[3] Superoxide dismutase (SOD) disarms free radicals produced in the energy centers of the cells known as the mitochondria, thereby improving energy production and reducing free radical damage in the body. Like SOD, glutathione is a natural compound that is found in all your cells. It is a potent antioxidant that helps destroy harmful free radicals before they can do damage to your cells, tissues, and joints.

Celery essential oil also contains compounds known as phthalides, which are known to be antispasmodic, suggesting that the oil may help with muscle pain in which spasms are involved. However, little research has been done in this area.

HOW TO USE

Taking celery essential oil internally is the best way to reap the effects of this remedy. It counteracts acidity in the joints while alleviating inflammation, making it an excellent choice for any type of joint pain, such as arthritis, bursitis, and gout. Celery essential oil is also highly effective against muscular pain conditions like fibromyalgia.

Begin by taking one drop three times daily for the first day or two. Increase to two drops three times daily. If you're not a fan of the taste, put the drops in empty capsules and take with water or juice.

You can also apply undiluted celery essential oil to painful joints or muscles. If you have sensitive skin, dilute three to six drops in a teaspoon of carrier oil, such as fractionated coconut oil or apricot kernel oil, before applying to sore muscles and joints.

SAFETY CONSIDERATIONS

While some sources indicate a possible skin sensitivity due to celery essential oil's furanocoumarin content, I haven't seen any studies that support the claim. If you're spending time outdoors or in a tanning bed, you may want to err on the side of caution. Keep celery essential oil out of reach of children. If you are pregnant, nursing, or under a doctor's care, consult your physician prior to use. Avoid contact with eyes, ears, and sensitive areas. Choose a product that is free of pesticides, as celery and celery seeds tend to be heavily sprayed crops.

SUPER HEALTH BONUS

Celery essential oil is also beneficial for poor digestion and digestive disorders, so don't be surprised if you notice an improvement in your digestion as well as your pain levels when using this potent natural medicine.

Cayenne and Other Chilies
(*Capsicum annum* L.)

When it comes to pain, turning up the heat can be the key to success. While some people wrongly believe the myth that chilies aggravate inflammation, research shows that they can actually reduce inflammation.

Pain is your body's way of letting you know that something is wrong. It does not only occur in localized areas; rather, it travels by way of the spinal cord and nervous system, sending pain messages to the brain. Intercepting these pain signals can be an effective strategy for alleviating pain. Research shows that capsaicin, one of the effective ingredients in cayenne and other chilies, intercepts such signals, blocking the transmission of pain in the skin. That's why so many anti-inflammatory ointments and creams contain high-concentration topical capsaicin,[1] which works against pain by depleting a brain messenger known as substance P, which is a pain neurotransmitter, in the area in which it is applied. Substance P transmits pain signals from the nerves in the skin through the spinal cord to the brain, where it is registered as pain. There is a link between high levels of substance P and many pain conditions.[2]

While some drugs like local anesthetics reduce substance P in the location where they are injected or applied, products made with cayenne, chilies, and capsaicin reduce pain but without interfering with perception of touch, temperature, or pressure in the affected areas.[3] In many studies, a topical cream or ointment containing 0.025 to 0.075 percent capsaicin was found to be helpful in treating arthritis; joint, muscle, and nerve pain; skin conditions involving pain, such as psoriasis and shingles; diabetic neuropathy; and postmastectomy pain. Capsaicin cream may also be effective in reducing pain in the extremely painful condition known as trigeminal neuralgia, which affects the nerves in the face. In these studies, participants applied the cream three times daily to yield results, so don't give up on capsaicin creams and ointments prematurely.

Not only does capsaicin deplete substance P when applied topically, but it is also a potent natural anti-inflammatory compound when ingested. Of course, I'm not talking about ingesting capsaicin creams or ointments. I'm referring to going to the source of the capsaicin and including more chilies in your diet. According to a study published in the *Cochrane Database of Systematic Reviews*, researchers found that eating cayenne peppers is beneficial for low back pain.[4]

HOW TO USE

Choose a topical cream or ointment that is free of synthetic and petrochemical ingredients and contains 0.025 to 0.075 percent capsaicin. Apply the cream to painful areas three times daily for at least a week. Discontinue use if you experience skin irritation or allergic reaction.

You can also choose a cayenne tincture. A typical dose is 0.25 to 1 milliliter, three times daily. One dropperful usually contains 1 milliliter of tincture.

To make an infusion (herbal tea), pour one cup of boiling water over one-half to one teaspoon of ground cayenne and allow to infuse for ten minutes. Drink three times daily for at least a week for best results.

Add fresh or dried cayenne or other chilies to your diet and continue to use on an ongoing basis for best results. It's not enough to eat a spicy meal on a periodic basis, although it may help with short-term pain relief. It is better to add cayenne, habanero, jalapeño, Thai bird, or other chilies to your favorite meals; ideally, make one meal a day a spicy one. You can add the chilies to soups, stews, curries, and other foods to ramp up the heat and the pain-alleviating properties.

SAFETY CONSIDERATIONS

When it comes to ingesting cayenne or other chilies, a little goes a long way. Some chilies are much hotter than others, so it is a good idea to start slowly and gradually build your tolerance. Keep in mind that the seeds and inner membranes of fresh chilies are the hottest parts, so don't use them if you're just starting to add chilies to your diet, or use them in small amounts at first. Wear gloves while chopping chilies or thoroughly wash your hands with soap after chopping. Avoid chopping chilies yourself if you suffer from asthma, since the fumes can trigger an attack. Avoid using if you have an ulcer.

I'm not aware of any side effects or drug interactions with cayenne. You may experience warmth in the area where capsaicin-based creams or ointments are applied to the skin.

SUPER HEALTH BONUS

Research from as early as the 1960s proves that ingesting cayenne or chilies may help improve blood circulation, particularly in the gastrointestinal tract, allowing foods that are ingested along with cayenne or other chilies to be assimilated faster and more readily.[5]

Clove Essential Oil
(*Eugenia caryophyllata*)

Imagine a spice so impressive that dangerous shipping expeditions and even wars were waged to ensure access to it. Cloves, and the oil extracted from them, have a rich and mysterious history that dates back to nearly four thousand years ago—their first known use was in 1721 BC.[1] As early as 226 BC, the Chinese chewed cloves before speaking to the emperor. In the sixteenth century, the Spanish explorer Ferdinand Magellan even risked his life to bring back a ship full of cloves and nutmeg to his mother country—a monumental feat, considering that cloves were worth more than gold at the time.

While ancient populations may have lacked the scientific technology and research to support their views, observation and a lengthy history of use ensured their knowledge of the healing spice. Clove is a powerful antioxidant that helps counter disease-causing and tissue-damaging free radicals.[2] It is a broad-spectrum antiseptic, fighting bacteria and viruses alike.[3] This may not sound relevant to our discussion about pain, but some conditions like arthritis have been linked to a possible bacterial infection[4] (which you can read more about in chapter 3).

Clove essential oil is a great natural remedy for joint pain. Clove oil contains a naturally occurring compound called eugenol, which is known for its anti-pain properties and is especially helpful for rheumatoid arthritis and osteoarthritis, as well as gout and fibromyalgia. Clove even improves circulation, which is often reduced due to swelling and inflammation.

Perhaps clove essential oil is best known for its ability to alleviate toothaches and other types of dental or oral pain, making it a common ingredient in natural toothpaste and mouthwash. If you suffer from cold sores, you'll want to make friends with clove essential oil. Research published in the *Journal of Dentistry* found that clove essential oil was as effective as the drug benzocaine for alleviating topical pain, such as the pain of cold sores.[5] Additionally, clove essential oil is often added to liniments and massage oils, since eugenol can be absorbed through the skin.

HOW TO USE

Dilute three to six drops of clove essential oil in one teaspoon of fractionated coconut or apricot kernel oil. Apply topically to sore joints or muscles, or for general achiness, on a daily basis, preferably two to three times daily, for best results. You can also apply the oil blend to cold sores or sore or sensitive teeth, or for dental pain. If you're using clove oil in your mouth, choose one that is suitable for internal use, since it is absorbed through the mucous membranes. Most essential oils on the market are not pure enough for this purpose, so you'll want to shop around for one that specifies internal use.

SAFETY CONSIDERATIONS

Because pure essential oil of cloves is quite concentrated and therefore highly potent, you'll need to dilute it in a carrier oil like apricot kernel or sweet almond oil prior to use. Just a few drops of clove oil per teaspoon of carrier oil makes an excellent natural and effective joint liniment. However, if you have sensitive skin, it may not be right for you.

Undiluted clove oil may cause skin irritation. Use with caution during pregnancy. Discontinue use if you experience any skin irritation. Avoid contact with eyes. Do not use in the ears.

SUPER HEALTH BONUS

If you suffer from diabetes, you'll be thrilled to know that research published in the *Journal of Medicinal Food* found that clove extracts were as effective as insulin in their initial tests on blood sugar levels.[6] Of course, that doesn't mean you should stop using insulin, as the result of stopping insulin can be fatal. It means that additional research is needed on the potential blood sugar support that cloves can offer those suffering from diabetes, but regular use may be helpful.

Copaiba Essential Oil

(*Copaifera reticulata, Copaifera officinalis, Copaifera coriacea, Copaifera langsdorffii*)

The vast jungles of the Amazon rain forest house some of the greatest diversity on the planet, including 3,000 species of fish, 1,300 species of birds, 430 species of amphibians, 380 species of reptiles, and an astonishing 40,000 species of plants.[1] Due to this incredible abundance of life, it is no wonder that some of the best plant-based remedies originate in this mysterious part of the world. In the canopy of the forest, the copaiba (pronounced co-pie-EE-ba) is one of the most exciting trees to rear its towering head, growing to around one hundred feet tall.

Traditional spiritual and physical healers of the region have used the resin from the copaiba tree for pain, for disorders of the urinary tract (including bladder and kidney infections), as a topical anti-inflammatory agent for a wide variety of skin disorders, as a gargle for sore throats and tonsillitis, and as a treatment for incontinence, stomach ulcers, syphilis, tetanus, bronchitis, herpes, tuberculosis, and more.[2]

In 1625, copaiba resin was recorded by Europeans and incorporated into their medicine when early Jesuit travelers brought it back from the New World under the label of Jesuit's balsam. In the early nineteenth century, copaiba was reported in a medical journal for its potential benefit in treating bronchitis.[3] Then, for around two hundred years, there was almost no mention of copaiba within medical journals. In the last several years, however, it is almost as though Western medicine has "rediscovered" copaiba, as a growing body of research begins to reveal what the indigenous peoples of South America have known for many years: that copaiba has widespread health benefits and is a potent, affordable, natural, nonaddictive painkiller.

Before diving into the many anti-pain and anti-inflammatory benefits of copaiba and how to use this powerful natural remedy, you may want to take a quick peek at the endocannabinoid system of the body, since that is the main way that copaiba interacts with the brain to yield its powerful results.

The Endocannabinoid System Holds the Key

It seems that the main reason for copaiba's many health benefits is its ability to interact with the powerful endocannabinoid system (ECS).[4] Most people have never heard of the ECS, having been taught only about the body's other systems: circulatory, digestive, endocrine (hormones and glands), integumentary (skin), lymphatic, muscular, nervous, reproductive, respiratory, skeletal, and urinary.[5] However, if you have looked into the healing benefits of marijuana, you are most likely already somewhat familiar with the ECS, since it is the system that interacts with cannabinoids like those found in cannabis. Since the discovery of cannabinoid receptors in the brain and nervous system, immune system, digestive tract, and many of the body's major organs, scientists have determined that there is an endocannabinoid system through which all of these receptors and cannabinoids work.[6] It has been called "a bridge between body and mind."[7]

There are two types of cannabinoid receptors: CB1 and CB2. CB1 receptors are found in the brain and nervous system, while CB2 receptors are primarily found in the digestive tract and immune system. They control a wide variety of functions in the body, including appetite, nausea, memory and cognitive functioning, reward, pressure in the eyes, and pain and discomfort, as well as the glands and hormones.[8]

There are three main cannabinoids: tetrahydrocannabinol (THC), cannabidiol (CBD), and beta-caryophyllene (BCP). You may recall that we reviewed these cannabinoids in chapter 5 in our discussion on cannabis. THC, the main psychoactive ingredient in marijuana, makes people feel "high" because it works on the CB1 receptors in the brain. CBD and BCP, also found in marijuana, are not psychoactive but have potent anti-pain and other effects on the body.

Copaiba contains high concentrations of BCP, which works exclusively on the CB2 receptors and gives copaiba its far-reaching effects without some of the unwanted ones that can come from other cannabinoids.[9]

Copaiba is quickly becoming best known for its ability to alleviate pain and inflammation, as a growing body of research showcases its impressive benefits. An animal study published in the *Journal of Cellular Biochemistry* found that copaiba demonstrated potent anti-inflammatory activity throughout the body and also reduced the number of free radicals that tend to be involved in the degradation of joints in arthritic conditions.[10]

In another study published in *Complementary Therapy in Clinical Practice*, researchers conducted a daily hand massage on people with arthritis in their hands using copaiba and a blend of oils with the product name Deep Blue. They reported a 50 percent decrease in pain scores.[11]

Copaiba also supports the health of the cardiovascular, immune, digestive, and respiratory systems; it acts as an antioxidant that helps destroy harmful disease-causing free radicals, while calming anxiety and supporting the nervous system. It is reported to help clear skin and reduce the appearance of blemishes.[12]

Copaiba essential oil is a powerful natural remedy that can be used in the treatment of a wide range of health conditions, including abdominal discomfort, arthritis and joint pain, burns, dental and oral pain, digestive pain, endometriosis, gout, heel spurs, inflammation, ligament and tendon pain, muscle pain or cramps, neuropathy and nerve pain, glaucoma or ocular pain and pressure (pressure in the eyes), plantar fasciitis, premenstrual syndrome (PMS) pain, sore throat, and tendonitis.

HOW TO USE

There are many ways to use copaiba essential oil, including diffusing it or mixing it with water and spraying into the air for the purpose of inhalation; diluting one to two drops of it in a small amount of carrier oil and applying topically to skin or other painful areas; or ingesting it for pain management or as part of a treatment for conditions like cancer or brain disease. It can also be mixed with honey to soothe sore throats and coughs.

SAFETY CONSIDERATIONS

Most copaiba essential oils on the market are not suitable for ingestion. Use only copaiba products that clearly indicate their suitability for internal use or that include the word *dose* on the bottle.

Make sure you select a high-quality, pure, undiluted copaiba essential oil. While you may end up diluting the oils yourself, most of the oils on the market are diluted with less-than-desirable carrier oils. High-quality oils cost more than the cheap varieties on the market but are worth the increased price. Cheap copaiba essential oil is adulterated with solvents used during the extraction process or toxic pesticides used in the growing process of the herbs from which the oils are extracted, and should therefore not be consumed.

Always conduct a forty-eight-hour test patch on a small, inconspicuous part of your skin to determine whether you have any sensitivity to the essential oils. Discontinue use if you experience any skin sensitivity. As with all essential oils, use copaiba with caution and under the advice of a qualified natural health practitioner during pregnancy or in the treatment of any health condition.[13]

Some companies may cut down the copaiba trees to extract the oil, thereby potentially destroying the delicate rain forest. Choose a product whose manufacturer taps the trees similar to the way that maple trees are tapped and does not overtap the trees, to ensure the life of the trees.

SUPER HEALTH BONUS

Because of copaiba's interaction with the endocannabinoid system, it also holds promise for the treatment of brain diseases like Parkinson's and Alzheimer's. It appears to work against Parkinson's disease through its ability to protect the nervous system from damage. A preliminary study published in the medical journal *Biomedicine & Pharmacotherapy* found that copaiba's effects on the CB2 receptors might help protect brain and nervous system cells involved with dopamine production and regulation.[14] In a study exploring the effects of copaiba on brain cells and Alzheimer's disease, researchers found that copaiba provided marked antioxidant, anti-inflammatory, and nerve- and brain-cell protecting abilities. The researchers also found that copaiba prevented the destruction of a brain hormone known as acetylcholine, whose deficiency has been linked to Alzheimer's.[15]

The endocannabinoid system is believed by many natural health professionals to hold the key to the future treatment of a wide range of diseases, including mood and anxiety disorders, movement disorders such as Parkinson's and Huntington's disease, neuropathic pain, multiple sclerosis, spinal cord injury, cancer, atherosclerosis, heart attacks, stroke, hypertension, glaucoma, obesity and metabolic syndrome, and osteoporosis.[16] As such, BCP found in copaiba may also hold promise in the treatment of a wide variety of health conditions. Additional research will determine whether this holds true for copaiba.

Devil's Claw

(*Harpagophytum procumbens*)

At first glance at this herb's name, you may be hesitant to use it. While devil's claw may sound a bit daunting, it is worth considering if you suffer from joint or back pain. And rest assured that "devil's claw" is only a moniker for the claw-like shape of the large fruit grown on this plant, not an indication of any potential threat it might pose to you.

Traditionally used by many herbalists in the treatment of arthritis, back pain, and other inflammatory conditions, devil's claw tends to work quickly to alleviate both pain and inflammation. Devil's claw may be used for the treatment of degenerative disorders of the musculoskeletal system, according to Germany's Commission E.[1] The Commission E Monographs are a compilation of the safety and effectiveness of herbs, showcasing those that have been approved by the German Ministry of Health.

Multiple studies demonstrate the herb's effectiveness on knee and hip osteoarthritis due to its ability to improve movement and reduce pain and crepitus.[2] Crepitus is any type of abnormal sound in the joints, including cracking, creaking, grating, or grinding.[3] In research published in the medical journal *Phytomedicine*, devil's claw was also found to be effective for low back and hip pain.[4] Research shows that devil's claw works on several levels: it inhibits substances that degrade joints and tissues, protects joints from damage, and reduces pain and inflammation.[5]

HOW TO USE

Devil's claw contains many active compounds, including harpagide, harpagoside, kaempferol, chlorogenic acid, cinnamic acid, luteolin, oleanolic acid, and procumbide. However, research published in the *Journal of Ethnopharmacology* found that the herb's effectiveness drops when extracts of specific compounds found in devil's claw are used independently.[6] It is best to take the whole plant, rather than just specific compounds like harpagoside, in capsule, tablet, or tincture form. Additional research published in the medical journal *Planta Medica* found that harpagoside taken on its own did not have the desired anti-inflammatory effect that devil's claw has.[7] If you choose capsules or tablets that contain standardized harpagosides, then you'll want to follow the package directions for the strength of the product you select; however, I think whole-herb products are safer and more effective.

The dose of devil's claw capsules and tablets tends to vary, so you should consult the package directions for the product you select, but it is typically two to three capsules or tablets, three times daily. If you're suffering from chronic pain like arthritis, you may want to take higher doses for arthritis than most devil's claw supplement packages recommend. A typical amount for arthritis is 2,500 milligrams of the whole plant daily, taken in divided doses. You can take this supplement with food or on an empty stomach, although some people find that taking any supplements on an empty stomach causes stomach upset. If you are among them, simply take this herb with food.

If you're using an alcohol extract, known as a tincture, a typical dose is 1 to 2 milliliters (a dropperful is 1 milliliter, or approximately thirty drops), three times daily.

If you're taking devil's claw as a tea, add one-half to one teaspoon of dried devil's claw per cup of water. Bring it to a boil and simmer for forty-five minutes. Drink one cup, three times daily. The mixture can also be made in advance and stored in the refrigerator for up to four days.

Many preparations of devil's claw are cut with a less expensive species known as *Harpagophytum zeyheri*. Be sure that the product you select contains *Harpagophytum procumbens*, not zeyheri.

SAFETY CONSIDERATIONS

Devil's claw might increase the effects of medications that reduce blood clotting, such as warfarin, so be sure to work with a knowledgeable doctor before taking these together. In some cases, people may be able to reduce their dose of warfarin while taking devil's claw, but you should be monitored by a physician if using devil's claw in conjunction with warfarin, since I don't recommend taking them together. Other medications that may interact with devil's claw include amitriptyline, celecoxib, diclofenac, glipizide, ibuprofen, losartan, meloxicam, and piroxicam, so check with your doctor or pharmacist if you are taking any of these drugs or any other medications.[8] Avoid using devil's claw if you are pregnant or have gallstones or an ulcer.

SUPER HEALTH BONUS

In a preliminary animal study published in the medical journal *Phytotherapy Research*, scientists found that devil's claw helped reduce the free radical damage, inflammation, and faulty immune response linked to the serious inflammatory bowel condition known as colitis, suggesting the herb may have potential in the disease's prevention and treatment.[9]

Eyebright

(*Euphrasia officinalis*)

You might not expect to see an herb named eyebright in a book about pain, but when it comes to painful eyes, whether due to glaucoma, conjunctivitis (pink eye), seasonal allergies, or any type of inflammation of the mucous membranes or tissue surrounding the eyes, eyebright is hard to beat.

It is an herb that has been used for centuries and possibly millennia for the treatment of eye problems, including eye irritation linked to allergies. A small but growing body of research demonstrates what our ancient ancestors knew and modern herbalists have experienced: eyebright works in the treatment of eye pain and inflammation, as well as oversensitivity to light.[1] Research published in the *Balkan Medical Journal* confirmed eyebright's anti-inflammatory activity and demonstrated that it also helped regulate overactive immune activity that may be damaging or painful to the eyes.[2]

Research published in the *Journal of Photochemistry and Photobiology* found that eye drops made from eyebright and chamomile were helpful to reduce free radicals in the eyes and the resulting eye damage and inflammation linked to ultraviolet-B (UVB) radiation.[3] Another study published in the *Journal of Alternative and Complementary Medicine* assessed the effect of eyebright eye drops on sixty-five people with eye irritation to determine the herb's effectiveness. The researchers found that the eye drops had a significant effect on the burning pain and redness of study participants. Fifty-three people (81.5 percent) had a complete recovery and eleven others (17 percent) had significant improvement. Additionally, there were no serious adverse events observed during the trial.[4]

It is unlikely that eyebright would be effective for other types of pain, but it is an excellent choice when dealing with eye pain. While I haven't seen any studies of its effect on eye pain linked to migraines, I have personally experienced some improvement in this regard.

HOW TO USE

Eyebright is available as a dry herb, tea, alcohol extract (tincture), and eye drops. To make the tea, steep one teaspoon of the dry herb or eyebright tea bag in one cup of boiled water for at least ten minutes. While the taste is mild, if you're not a fan, you can add a teaspoon of peppermint or a peppermint herbal tea bag to make it more palatable. Drink three cups daily for the best results. Alternatively, brew the herbal tea and soak a clean washcloth in it. Wring out and apply as a compress to painful eyes (closed eyes, of course) once the cloth is warm but not hot. Reapply as necessary for pain relief.

Take thirty drops of eyebright tincture orally, two or three times daily. Follow the package instructions for capsules. *Do not put the herb or alcohol tincture in your eyes.* Choose only eyebright eye drops specifically made for this purpose. Follow package directions for the eye drops.

SAFETY CONSIDERATIONS

I'm unaware of any safety issues or drug interactions with eyebright.

SUPER HEALTH BONUS

As its name suggests, this herb helps keep eyes bright and healthy and helps address the eye symptoms linked to allergies or infections: itchy eyes, redness, swollen eyes, and eye irritation.

Fennel Essential Oil

(*Foeniculum vulgare*)

Fennel was used as food and medicine in ancient India, Egypt, Greece, and Rome. Ancient Roman warriors used fennel because they believed it gave them the strength they needed for battle.[1] While not technically a pain remedy (many herbal experts would be surprised to find it among these pages), fennel essential oil can reduce premenstrual pain and cramps.

In an animal study published in the *Journal of Ethnopharmacology*, researchers found that fennel essential oil was effective in reducing the intensity and frequency of menstrual abdominal contractions linked to inflammation-causing compounds known as prostaglandins.[2]

Another study published in the *Iranian Journal of Nursing and Midwifery Research* assessed the effectiveness of fennel, along with vitamin E, in comparison to ibuprofen.[3] While both fennel and ibuprofen showed effectiveness against pain, fennel demonstrated greater effectiveness, particularly one to two hours after administration, and its overall ability to alleviate pain was superior to that of ibuprofen, without any of the side effects linked to the drug, which include nausea, dyspepsia, diarrhea, fatigue, and liver damage.

The scientists who conducted this study believe fennel's analgesic effect may be largely due to its anethole content, since this ingredient is best known for its antispasmodic actions, making it an excellent choice for menstrual cramps. Additionally, anethole joins to the body's dopamine receptors to decrease pain.

Though the study used an alcohol extract of the herb, oil extracts of fennel also contain anethole, making the use of fennel essential oil a good way to reap the benefits of the herb. While both can be used internally, the essential oil may be preferable because it can be combined with a carrier oil like fractionated coconut oil or apricot kernel oil and rubbed over the lower abdomen to help ease premenstrual and menstrual cramps.

HOW TO USE

Fennel essential oil can be diffused, used topically, and, when a pure enough extract is used, taken internally, following safety precautions, of course (see page 25 for more information about using essential oils internally, and see the following paragraph).

If using fennel essential oil internally, take one drop three times daily on your tongue or in an empty capsule. You can also add a drop to a glass of water or juice three times daily. Fennel has a pleasing licorice taste, but obviously if you're not a fan of licorice, you may prefer to ingest it in an empty capsule to avoid tasting it. You can take fennel when you are menstruating or suffering from cramps, but the best results are typically achieved when it is used throughout the month.

Additionally, apply diluted fennel essential oil over your abdominal area once or twice daily, not just during your periods but throughout the month.

SAFETY CONSIDERATIONS

Keep in mind that not all fennel essential oil is suitable for internal use. Choose a reputable brand with third-party laboratory testing that demonstrates its purity. Also, check the label of the product you select. If it doesn't include the word *dose*, then it is not suitable for internal use and should not be ingested.

Dilute fennel essential oil for skin application and patch test before using. It may cause skin sensitivity. Use with caution during pregnancy and with children under the age of five. It is not for use with epilepsy or seizures.

SUPER HEALTH BONUS

Fennel is beneficial for digestive health, so don't be surprised if you experience improved digestion, reduced abdominal bloating, and less nausea, flatulence, and constipation.

Feverfew

(*Tanacetum parthenium*)

Most people don't believe me when I tell them that I lived in two semi-arid desert regions in Canada where the temperatures routinely exceeded 100 degrees Fahrenheit or 40 degrees Celsius in the summer. Even most Canadians don't believe that there are deserts in Canada, but the hundreds of small cacti on the stone walls and mountainside on the property where I lived proved it.

Unlike some desert regions that don't support much plant life other than cacti, one of the areas I lived in was slightly damper than the other and, as a result, had tremendous botanical diversity. On that property I found the lovely, small, daisy-like plant known as feverfew growing in my gardens and on the hillside.

One of the things I've learned over the years of studying herbalism and natural medicine is that plants that survive in extreme conditions, such as drought, high altitude, heat, or cold, tend to have higher amounts of healing compounds called phytochemicals, which literally means "plant chemicals." The compounds that ensure the plants' survival in these harsh conditions also offer healing properties when we use them. Feverfew, which can grow in hot conditions with little water, is a most impressive healer and all-around great pain reliever. Not only does it have analgesic properties that can reduce the pain of migraines or arthritis, but it also reduces inflammation and acts as an antispasmodic to help alleviate menstrual cramps. Well-constructed studies of feverfew have also demonstrated it could significantly reduce the prevalence of migraines,[1] a particularly excruciating form of headache that is characterized by knifing pain in one eye.

I routinely hear from people who tell me that feverfew doesn't work, so I proceed to ask them how they took it, and inevitably find that they popped some feverfew pills or drank some feverfew tea when their migraine was particularly bad. Because the herb does not offer immediate relief, most people assume it doesn't work. In reality, feverfew is remarkably effective against migraines, but not when used in this manner.

Feverfew works best against migraines when taken regularly as a preventive measure. Preventive use not only reduces the incidence of migraines but reduces the incidence and severity of headaches in chronic sufferers. Taking feverfew as one takes migraine medications or over-the-counter pain relievers, *after* the onset of pain, is rarely effective.

Feverfew may also help with the painful neurological condition known as neuropathy. *Neuropathy* is a general term used to describe disorders of the nervous system that cause pain, weakness, and numbness. It is a possible side effect of cancer chemotherapy. In a study published in the journal *Phytomedicine*, researchers found that feverfew was as effective as the drug gabapentin (an antiepileptic drug that has also been found to alleviate neuropathic pain).[2] Interestingly, the scientists who conducted the study found significant improvement in nerve-related pain when an extract of the flowers was used but none when the leaves were used, yet many feverfew products are made primarily from the leaves. The feverfew flower extract reduced neuropathy caused by the chemotherapy drug oxaliplatin and the antiviral drug dideoxycytidine.

Feverfew may also be beneficial for arthritis due to its anti-inflammatory properties.

HOW TO USE

The aerial parts of the plant (those parts that are above the ground—leaves, flowers, and stems) are used in herbal medicine. You can make tea from one teaspoon of the dried herb per cup of boiled water. Pour the water over the herb and allow to steep for at least ten to fifteen minutes. Drink three times daily.

You can also take a feverfew tincture. The typical dose is thirty drops, three times daily, for at least a month. Tinctures prepared from fresh plant material are preferable to those made from the dried plant; however, this information is rarely disclosed on product labels, so it may not be possible to discern between them.

Alternatively, the recommended dosage is 25 to 125 milligrams daily of a standardized leaf and flower extract containing a minimum of 0.2 percent parthenolide. Higher doses (up to 2 grams daily) may be required for a day or two for the treatment of a migraine or other inflammatory condition.[3]

If you're suffering from neuropathy, you may find herbal preparations made exclusively from the flowers to be superior to whole-herb products.

SAFETY CONSIDERATIONS

Using feverfew requires some caution. If you are allergic to ragweed, you may also be allergic to feverfew. Pregnant or nursing women should avoid feverfew. The prescription blood thinner warfarin can interact with feverfew, so it is best not to take both together. Additionally, if you routinely take over-the-counter painkillers, it is best to skip feverfew. Also avoid taking it for a couple of weeks prior to undergoing surgery. Consult your physician prior to use.

SUPER HEALTH BONUS

Not only will feverfew help your headaches, migraines, menstrual pain, or neuropathy but it may also help if you suffer from allergies. That's because feverfew has demonstrated the ability to reduce histamine secretion by the body, which is the body's response to allergens and is responsible for the many symptoms linked to allergies.[4] Reducing histamine secretion will likely reduce allergy symptoms like congestion, itchy eyes, and sneezing. Of course, if you have ragweed allergies, you probably won't reap the antihistamine benefits of feverfew and may have an allergic response, so the herb is best avoided.

Frankincense Essential Oil
(*Boswellia frereana, Boswellia serrata*)

I f I was stranded on a deserted island and could choose only one essential oil to have with me, I might select either copaiba or frankincense, since both oils are versatile and powerful healing remedies. Frankincense was a part of the spiritual rituals of ancient Egyptians, Babylonians, Persians, Hebrews, Greeks, and Romans, and of course, it is considered a precious gift according to Christian beliefs—the perfect gift from three wise men. And, because it was so often burned for its purification purposes, even frankincense char was used by ancient Egyptian women as their characteristic black eyeliner, long before chemical eyeliner products became commonplace.

In addition to its ancient spiritual and cosmetic uses, frankincense offers relief from pain and inflammation. Frankincense is better known among herbal medicine practitioners as boswellia, or *Boswellia serrata*, and is beneficial for both osteoarthritis and rheumatoid arthritis, as well as many other painful conditions. In an animal study published in the *Asian Pacific Journal of Tropical Medicine*, researchers investigated the analgesic effect of frankincense by administering its crude extract, essential oil, and various subfractions of the extract orally to mice in pain tests. While animal studies are often criticized, their lack of placebo effect gives them an advantage when testing pain remedies. In this study, the scientists determined the validity of frankincense and its analgesic effects for alleviating arthritis and muscle aches and pains, as well as stomach discomfort.[1]

In a double-blind study published in the medical journal *Phytotherapy Research*, scientists compared a frankincense supplement with a placebo in people with knee osteoarthritis and found significant improvements in the frankincense group. The frankincense reduced the amount of a C-reactive protein, a highly inflammatory compound that is a potential inflammation marker for osteoarthritis. The people taking the frankincense supplement also demonstrated marked improvement in the health of their knee joints.[2]

A study published in the *European Review for Medical and Pharmacological Sciences* assessing a supplement that combined frankincense with ginger and glucosamine had similar results for people suffering from knee osteoarthritis. The researchers found that study participants had significant improvements in pain and a reduction in markers of inflammation after one-, three-, and six-month milestones.[3]

Other research published in the medical journal *Musculoskeletal Surgery* found that frankincense, along with turmeric and standard drug-based analgesics, significantly reduced the pain linked to shoulder surgery and damaged rotator cuff tendons in the shoulders.[4]

Frankincense is suitable for more than just joint pain. A study published in the *European Review for Medical and Pharmacological Sciences* found that the natural remedy was also effective for the abdominal pain linked to irritable bowel syndrome (IBS),[5] which is great news if you're one of the 12 percent of Americans who suffer from abdominal discomfort, bloating, irregular bowel movements, and alternating constipation or diarrhea linked to the condition.[6]

While frankincense may be beneficial for many other pain disorders, there is currently insufficient research beyond musculoskeletal and brain health. Given its many benefits and low likelihood of side effects, it is certainly worth considering for other conditions. After witnessing frankincense's widespread healing abilities, I coined the statement "When in doubt, frank it out" in reference to the oil's versatility and ability to help almost any physical health or emotional imbalance.

HOW TO USE

While frankincense is available in many herbal preparations, I prefer a frankincense essential oil suitable for internal use to ensure rapid absorption and, as a result, faster healing effects. You can also diffuse the oil or apply it diluted in a carrier oil like fractionated coconut oil to painful areas, but I find internal use to be most effective for pain conditions. Take three drops at a time, three times daily. Of course, most types of pain also respond well to direct application of the oil to the affected area.

SAFETY CONSIDERATIONS

Be sure the product you choose has been approved for internal use, as most products are not pure enough for this purpose. Frankincense is safe for undiluted (neat) topical use provided a pure product is used; dilute for sensitive skin.

SUPER HEALTH BONUS

Don't be surprised if you experience an improvement in your moods while using frankincense essential oil for pain. In a study published in the *Journal of Psychopharmacology*, a natural compound found in frankincense was found to have antidepressant qualities. The compound, known as incensole acetate (IA), was found to regulate hormones secreted by the hypothalamus, pituitary, and adrenal glands. The hypothalamus and pituitary glands are located in the brain and are involved in mood regulation, while the adrenal glands sit atop the kidneys and help address stress in the body. The researchers concluded that frankincense has potential as a novel treatment for depression.[7] Frankincense also contains compounds known as sesquiterpenes, which cross the blood-brain barrier and may help oxygenate the glands in the brain.[8]

Ginger Essential Oil and Herb
(*Zingiber officinale*)

When most people think of ginger, they probably think of ginger-bread or gingersnaps, but this herb is also one of my favorite natural remedies for alleviating pain and inflammation. Unlike some herbs that are suitable for a specific type of pain, ginger works on almost any type of pain. I say "almost," but it has worked well on all the types of pain for which I have used it, although obviously there may be other conditions with which I'm unfamiliar.

Ginger is extremely effective against muscle and joint pain, making it a great choice for anyone suffering from osteoarthritis, rheumatoid arthritis, fibromyalgia, or other forms of arthritis. Research published in the medical journal *Arthritis* compared ginger with cortisone and ibuprofen, both drugs that are used in the treatment of inflammatory conditions, and found that ginger was superior to ibuprofen at reducing inflammatory compounds known as cytokines and was equally as effective as cortisone. Unlike cortisone, however, ginger does not have a lengthy list of nasty side effects.[1]

In a study published in the journal *Arthritis and Rheumatism* of 261 people suffering from osteoarthritis of the knees, those who ingested ginger extract daily had a significant improvement in joint pain over those who received the placebo.[2]

A study published in the *Journal of Alternative and Complementary Medicine* compared ginger extract to the nonsteroidal anti-inflammatory drug (NSAID) diclofenac. Some study participants received a ginger extract while others received diclofenac. Both groups had similar reductions in pain, but the group taking the ginger extract had fewer gastrointestinal complaints than the drug group.[3]

In a study published in the medical journal *Arthritis*, scientists discovered that ginger was as effective as the anti-inflammatory cortisone drug betamethasone. It was also superior to ibuprofen in the same study. Ibuprofen did not work to reduce levels of inflammatory cytokines, while ginger was highly effective in this capacity.[4] Cytokines are compounds that are initially involved in immune reactions in the body but quickly become detrimental to healthy cells and tissues, so reducing them is a valuable strategy in addressing arthritis symptoms and joint damage.

While NSAIDs work on only one biochemical level in the body, ginger works on at least two mechanisms: it blocks the formation of pain-causing substances like prostaglandins and leukotrienes, and it breaks down inflammation and acidity in the fluid surrounding the joints.[5] Most drugs work only on the former mechanism and simply cannot compete with ginger for effectiveness against joint pain, particularly when ginger is used daily over months or years. In this time frame, ginger helps heal the joints, not just reduce pain.

In several other studies, ginger has been found to be more effective than ibuprofen without causing all the negative side effects that have been linked to ibuprofen use, like rashes, ringing in the ears, headaches, dizziness, drowsiness, abdominal pain, nausea, diarrhea, constipation, heartburn, stomach or intestinal ulcerations, impaired kidney function, and even death.

Compare the abbreviated drug side-effect list above to that of ginger, whose side effects are more energy, improved digestion, and a speedier metabolism in people who are overweight. Some people do experience occasional mild gastrointestinal irritation from its use, but for most people ginger actually benefits digestive health. And unlike pharmaceutical painkillers, ginger is not addictive. So ginger's track record of safety makes it a great choice for most conditions.

While there are many excellent recent studies on ginger's effectiveness, I particularly like an older one conducted by Dr. Krishna C. Srivastava, a world-renowned researcher of the therapeutic effects of spices. In one study, Dr. Srivastava gave patients suffering from rheumatoid arthritis, osteoarthritis, or muscle pain ginger powder daily for a period lasting a minimum of three months and tracked their progress for up to two and a half years. All the patients suffering from muscle pain had relief, and over 75 percent of rheumatoid arthritis and osteoarthritis sufferers had significant improvements in pain and swelling. None of the patients in this study had any negative side effects from ingesting ginger.[6] As if that wasn't impressive enough, Dr. Srivastava also found that ginger has antioxidant effects that break down existing inflammation and acidity in the fluid within the joints, which helps their healing.[7]

Its versatility, safety, and effectiveness are probably among the reasons why ginger has been used for thousands of years in Ayurvedic medicine in India as a natural anti-inflammatory food. Ginger is also one of the best herbs to address muscular or joint pain and inflammation (like that experienced by sufferers of fibromyalgia and arthritis).

HOW TO USE

The amount used in Dr. Srivastava's study was 5 grams of fresh ginger or one teaspoon of dried ginger, in divided doses throughout the day. Fresh or dried ginger can be added to stir-fries, curries, soups, noodle dishes, or vegetable dishes or made into tea.

To make a ginger tea, chop a two- to three-inch piece of fresh ginger, add it to a quart of water, and boil on the stove for thirty to sixty minutes. Add one to three drops of stevia to sweeten each cup of tea. Drink at least three cups daily for arthritic or muscle pain. You can also add an inch or two of fresh gingerroot to your juicer when making your favorite juices. You can make this beverage ahead of time and store in the fridge to drink up to three days later.

While eating ginger is quite helpful, sometimes you may need the faster, stronger relief that ginger capsules, tincture (alcohol extract), or essential oil can provide. If you're using a powdered ginger supplement, take four capsules at once, three times daily, until you begin to experience an improvement in pain, then reduce your dose to three capsules twice daily. If you have bouts of pain, you can return to the higher dose for a few days and then drop back down to the lower maintenance dose. Note: this refers to a whole, dried ginger supplement, not an extract of gingerols or other compounds found in ginger.

Alternatively, you can take a dropperful of tincture three times daily to start experiencing pain relief.

You can also apply ginger essential oil topically to the skin, diluted in a carrier oil, since it stimulates circulation and is helpful for joint and muscle stiffness and pain.

In my experience, the most effective way to experience ginger's pain-relieving effects is to take ginger essential oil internally. It's too hot to use directly in the mouth, so I suggest using empty capsules and adding three drops of ginger essential oil. Take three to four times daily, or more, if necessary, for the first few days, but do not exceed twenty drops of essential oil total. That number includes any other essential oils you may be using internally.

SAFETY CONSIDERATIONS

Keep in mind that most ginger essential oil sold in pharmacies and department stores is not suitable for internal use and should be avoided. Choose a product that is designed for internal use and is free of toxic solvents and other unwanted ingredients. The company should be able to provide third-party laboratory testing. The product you select should also have the word *dose* on the label; otherwise, it is not pure enough for internal use. See page 23 for additional safety instructions on using essential oils.

Dilute ginger essential oil before applying topically. It may cause skin sensitivity. Discontinue use if you have a skin reaction.

SUPER HEALTH BONUS

A natural and gentle stimulant, ginger essential oil helps boost circulation, which warms the body and helps boost energy levels. Additionally, it improves digestion and metabolism, making it an excellent choice for anyone trying to lose weight.

Lavender Essential Oil

(*Lavandula angustifolia*)

Soon after I moved to British Columbia, Canada, I went for a leisurely drive to a town about an hour away, down a winding, scenic lakeside road with stunning vineyards scattered across the countryside. As I neared the end of the road, the intensely fragrant scent of lavender filled my senses, long before I could even *see* the flowers. I drove down a side road and traveled about a half mile through the rolling hillside before finally spotting the source of the heavenly aroma: the stunning silvery-green and violet-colored plants at a lavender farm. I felt immediately transported to a peaceful, relaxed state. How much was linked to the actual aromatic effects of lavender or the natural beauty of it in this lovely environment, I'll never know. Either way, it was an experience that I won't forget.

Lavender has been in use for at least 2,500 years, including for mummification and perfumery by the ancient Egyptians, Phoenicians, and Arabs. The flowers were infused in water in Roman baths, which led to the modern name for lavender (from the Latin *lavare*, which means "to wash"). Ancient Romans are also believed to have used lavender for cooking and for scenting the air. In ancient Rome, lavender flowers were so highly prized that a single pound was sold for the equivalent of a month of a farm worker's wages.[1] During the height of the Plague, glove makers scented their leatherware with lavender oil, which was believed to ward off the deadly infection.[2]

The oil extract of the delicate, lovely flowers of lavender provides a potent natural remedy that, while not specifically a pain remedy, can help address hormonal imbalances during a woman's menstrual cycle. A study published in the journal *BioPsychoSocial Medicine* found that inhaling the scent of lavender for ten minutes had a significant beneficial effect on the nervous system of women suffering from premenstrual symptoms and could decrease feelings of depression.[3] While the study focused on emotional pain, the hormonal imbalances that occur during a woman's period can also result in painful cramping.

Considering that chronic pain can result in depression, anxiety, or difficulty sleeping, not only for women during their menstrual periods but for anyone dealing with chronic pain, lavender can help address all of these issues.

In a study published in the medical journal *Complementary Therapies in Clinical Practice*, researchers found that when women inhaled two drops of lavender essential oil at three intervals during labor, they experienced a significant reduction in labor pain.[4]

Lavender's ability to affect the nervous system suggests it may also offer hope for those suffering from nerve pain linked to various pain conditions. In an animal study published in the medical journal *Frontiers in Pharmacology*, researchers found that lavender essential oil was effective in reducing neuropathy pain.[5] A recent study in the *Journal of Neuroimmunology* corroborated the earlier study, finding that lavender essential oil was effective in reducing chronic inflammation and neuropathy pain.[6]

Lavender essential oil is also showing promise in preliminary studies of its use for osteoarthritis pain. In research published in *Complementary Therapies in Clinical Practice*, scientists applied lavender essential oil to affected knees of study participants. The study found that the results were best both immediately and one week after continued use, but then tapered off.[7] More research needs to be conducted to determine the short- and long-term results of topically applied lavender essential oil for the management of painful osteoarthritic joints, but based on lavender's impressive safety record, it is worth considering for those suffering from osteoarthritis.

Lavender essential oil has traditionally been used to speed the healing and ease the pain of burns and wounds of all kinds, including those involving sunburn, fire, or scalding. The efficacy of these traditional uses have been verified by extensive research, including a study in the journal *Complementary Therapies in Clinical Practice* that showed that lavender essential oil reduced the recovery time needed after episiotomies linked to childbirth.[8] Additionally, research published in the journal *Phytotherapy Research* found that scientific and clinical data support the traditional uses of lavender essential oil.[9]

If you're suffering from hormone-related pain, nerve pain, or burns of any kind, it is worth considering lavender for your pain management protocol.

HOW TO USE

Lavender essential oil can be diffused in an aromatherapy diffuser, applied topically, or used internally. In my experience, while diffusing lavender essential oil works well to relax the nervous system, ease stress, and alleviate anxiety and depression, the best way to experience lavender's analgesic effects is to apply it topically to painful areas and deeply inhale the aroma at least a few times daily. Obviously, that's not possible for all types of pain, so diffusing may be a good option for some conditions.

SAFETY CONSIDERATIONS

Purchase lavender essential oil that is extracted from the lavender species *Lavandula angustifolia*. Most of the lavender oils on the market are made from cheaper varieties that do not yield the same therapeutic results. If you've selected pure, high-quality, therapeutic-grade lavender essential oil, it is likely safe to apply undiluted (neat) directly to your skin, unless you have highly sensitive skin. If you have sensitive skin, dilute one drop of lavender with five drops of a carrier oil like fractionated coconut or apricot kernel oil before applying. It is best to conduct a forty-eight-hour skin patch test on the inside of your wrist before applying to a more widespread area.

SUPER HEALTH BONUS

The *BioPsychoSocial Medicine* study mentioned earlier found that lavender decreased feelings of depression and confusion in female study participants. That's not surprising given lavender's ability to alleviate anxiety and depression. It was even found to be slightly more effective than an antidepressant drug in another study.[10] Lavender helps relax the nervous system, making it an effective insomnia remedy that promotes a deeper, more regenerative sleep at night. These benefits may be valuable for someone experiencing trouble sleeping, anxiety, depression, or the mental and emotional effects of chronic pain.

As an added bonus, lavender essential oil is a natural tick and mosquito repellent that can be added to your favorite unscented moisturizer before heading outdoors. For best results, you'll want to reapply every couple of hours if you're spending time outside.

Licorice Root

(*Glycyrrhiza glabra*)

Licorice root—the herb, not the candy—is one of my favorite herbs, not only because of its unique taste and profound healing powers but also because of its wide-reaching applications. While few people would ever consider licorice root a pain remedy, it offers excellent foundational support for many health conditions.

Licorice root contains natural cortisone-like substances that can help reduce the inflammation underlying many pain disorders and may prove useful in the long-term treatment and management of these conditions.

In a study published in the journal *Natural Product Communications*, scientists compared the anti-inflammatory capabilities of several herbs to those of ibuprofen. The scientists concluded that licorice proved even more effective than ibuprofen in alleviating the inflammation linked to arthritis.[1] Another study published in the *Journal of Agricultural and Food Chemistry* found that licorice was also helpful in the treatment of rheumatoid arthritis.[2]

Unlike drugs that can only either stimulate or reduce the function of an organ or organ system, licorice is one of the highly coveted herbs that are classified as adaptogens, meaning it can both increase *and* decrease outputs of the body to bring about balance, depending on what is needed. This makes the herb a valuable choice for painful autoimmune disorders in which an overactive immune system attacks the body's own tissues, such as rheumatoid arthritis, lupus, and the skin condition known as scleroderma.

Licorice works, at least in part, by resetting the body's glands. The adrenal glands, two small triangular-shaped glands that sit atop the kidneys, are vulnerable to stress from the pressures we face in our fast-paced modern world. The "adrenaline rush" many people get from driving themselves hard to excel or from extreme sports may seem great at the time, but over longer periods it can wear down the adrenal glands, causing a whole host of physical ailments, such as fatigue, poor digestion, sleep disorders, reduced or impaired immune system functioning, elevated blood sugar levels, and of course, pain and inflammation. The adrenal glands produce the body's own natural cortisone, but as the glands become depleted, they are no longer able to produce sufficient amounts to reduce inflammation in the body. Fortunately, licorice is one of the best herbs to restore the body's hypothalamus-pituitary-adrenal axis (the HPA axis), the part of the endocrine system that regulates the flow of adrenal outputs.

A study published in the medical journal *Pharmaceutical Biology* found that licorice works to reduce inflammation on multiple levels, including regulating cortisol production in the body and reducing free radicals and three other pain- or inflammation-causing compounds.[3] These abilities to regulate cortisol and decrease damaging compounds in the body are at least some of the reasons for licorice root's ability to help a large number of pain conditions.

Licorice also works by restoring gut health, which you learned about in chapter 3. In summary, there have been volumes of research linking the health of the gut to the health of the body, including pain conditions. Naturally-minded doctors recognize the value of restoring gut health with herbs that act as gentle, mild laxatives and also soothe the lining of the gut, both of which licorice root does. Licorice root reduces inflammation in the intestines and helps eliminate toxic waste in the bowels. Its role in protecting and healing damaged mucous membranes in the intestinal tract has been confirmed by hundreds of studies, according to Daniel B. Mowrey, author of *The Scientific Validation of Herbal Medicine*.[4] Licorice root may also help soothe pain in other regions of the body as well.

HOW TO USE

You can purchase premade licorice root tea bags. Drink three cups daily for up to three weeks. Alternatively, take thirty drops of licorice root tincture three times daily for up to three weeks. You can also purchase licorice supplements. Choose one that says "DGL" on the bottle, which stands for deglycyrrhizinated licorice. This means the manufacturer has removed a substance known as glycyrrhizin from the licorice, making it safer for use.

SAFETY CONSIDERATIONS

Because it is such a powerful herb, licorice can have harmful side effects if misused, so it is important to use it with care. Regardless of which type you select, be sure to discontinue its use after three weeks, since licorice can throw off the balance of minerals known as electrolytes when used for extended periods. Also, because many drugs interact with licorice, you should consult your physician or pharmacist to find out if any medications you may be taking interact with licorice root. Individuals with high blood pressure or kidney failure, as well as people taking heart medication, should avoid licorice. It should not be used in large quantities or for periods longer than a few weeks without the guidance of a qualified herbalist or medical practitioner.

SUPER HEALTH BONUS

While you're taking licorice to alleviate the inflammation underlying your pain condition, you might find that it also goes to work to help your health in other ways. That's especially true if you are suffering from cancer or trying to prevent it. Preliminary research published in the medical journal *Fitoterapia* suggested that the compound glabridin, found in licorice root, was able to prevent liver cancer genes from turning on.[5] In breast cancer, the cancer's own stem cells are believed to cause metastasis (cancer spreading to other parts of the body) and recurrence. In a study published in the journal *Molecular Carcinogenesis*, scientists found that glabridin could inhibit the functions of cancer stem cells. The scientists concluded that licorice root may be "a potential treatment strategy . . . [and a way to] enhance the effectiveness of breast cancer therapy."[6]

Marjoram Essential Oil and Herb

(*Origanum majorana*)

Marjoram, an herb that grows just over one foot tall, was used by the ancient Egyptians in skin care and perfumes. Known by a Greek word that means "joy of the mountains," marjoram was a symbol of happiness to ancient Greeks as well as Romans.[1] The women of ancient Greece infused oil with marjoram to use on their heads as a relaxant.[2] While the herb has had many uses throughout history, perhaps the first-century Greek physician Dioscorides was most famously aware of its inherent anti-pain properties when he made an ointment called amaricimum from marjoram to warm and strengthen the nerves.[3]

According to an animal study published in the *Journal of Ethnopharmacology*, researchers found that marjoram effectively relaxed muscles and alleviated abdominal pain.[4] And marjoram essential oil works regardless of whether the abdominal pain is hormonal in nature or due to another cause. In another study published in the *Journal of Obstetrics and Gynaecology Research*, scientists explored the effects of marjoram essential oil on painful periods in women. They found that marjoram essential oil reduced not only the menstrual pain and cramp- ing but also the duration of time women suffered from this condition, known as dysmenorrhea.[5]

In a study published in the *Journal of Alternative and Complementary Medicine*, researchers also found that marjoram essential oil, in conjunction with black pepper, lavender, and peppermint, reduced upper shoulder tension and significantly reduced neck pain.[6] Because many headaches and migraines originate in neck and shoulder tension, marjoram essential oil applied directly to these tight areas, as well as the back of the head at the base of the skull, can often be helpful.

Due to marjoram's ability to address muscle spasms and tightness while also alleviating pain, it may have wide-reaching applications, including for muscle sprains, muscle strains, gastrointestinal (GI) pain, neck pain, fibromyalgia, and upper, mid, or low back pain. It may also have applications for eye and nervous system–related pain.[7] Marjoram may also be helpful in the treatment of carpal tunnel syndrome, tendonitis, and arthritis.[8]

Marjoram contains many healing compounds, including several antioxidants—ursolic acid, carnosic acid, carnosol, hydroquinone, and rosmarinic acid—and numerous phenolic compounds, all of which help protect the body from free radical damage. This is particularly important in dealing with chronic inflammatory pain conditions, since they typically entail free radical damage to joints, muscles, tissues, or nerves.

HOW TO USE

While you can add marjoram to your vegetable, legume, meat, poultry, mushroom, or other dishes to boost their flavor and therapeutic value, you'll want to take it in a higher dose to fully benefit from its anti-pain and anti-inflammatory properties. You can supplement with the herb in capsules, taking three capsules of the whole herb with meals three times daily. If you're using a product in which any of the compounds have been standardized (meaning an active ingredient is added to a supplement to reach a certain percentage of the total product), follow package instructions for the product you select. Marjoram is also available in alcohol extracts, known as tinctures. The standard dosage is one dropperful, three times daily, but it is best to follow package instructions for the product you select.

I prefer marjoram essential oil, since it is concentrated and thus a convenient way to benefit from marjoram's therapeutic, anti-pain, and anti-inflammatory properties. You can take two to three drops of marjoram essential oil in an empty capsule, three times daily, provided that you select a high-quality essential oil with third-party laboratory testing to ensure purity.

Marjoram essential oil can also be diluted in a carrier oil such as fractionated coconut oil and applied directly to painful areas. See the following safety considerations for more information about ingestion and topical application.

SAFETY CONSIDERATIONS

Not all marjoram essential oils are suitable for ingestion. Actually, most of the marjoram oils on the market are not appropriate for internal use. As a result, you should use only ones that are clearly designated for internal use. This is easily identifiable on the label, which should include the word *dose* or *dosage*.

While the dose in the *Journal of Alternative and Complementary Medicine* study mentioned earlier was 4 percent marjoram essential oil in a cream base, most people can tolerate a higher dose than that. If you have sensitive skin, do not exceed 4 percent. Discontinue use if you have a skin reaction. Conduct a forty-eight-hour skin patch test prior to using more extensively. See page 23 for more information on using essential oils.

Avoid using marjoram essential oil or marjoram herb during the first trimester of pregnancy; use with caution or under a qualified health professional's direction during pregnancy or while nursing.

SUPER HEALTH BONUS

According to a study published in the journal *Natural Product Research*, a variety of marjoram known as pot marjoram or Greek oregano was as effective as DEET-based insecticides at repelling mosquitoes. Incidentally, marjoram is also highly effective at repelling ticks, making it an excellent choice when you're heading to wooded areas.[9]

Myrrh Essential Oil
(*Commiphora molmol, Commiphora myrrha*)

The resin from the small, thorny tree known as *Commiphora molmol* or *Commiphora myrrha*, myrrh has a lengthy tradition of use as incense, in meditation rituals, and in treating many ailments, from fighting infections to healing skin conditions. First recorded for medicinal use in AD 600 in Chinese medical literature during the Tang dynasty, myrrh also has origins as a gift from the three wise men in Christian biblical times.[1] Modern research is proving what the ancient populations seem to have known: that myrrh is a potent natural medicine and powerful pain reliever.

Research published in the journal *BioMed Research International* assessed the effects of a myrrh supplement on ninety-five women and eighty-nine men, ranging from eighteen to sixty years old, with a wide variety of pain conditions, including headaches, joint pain, muscle aches, low back pain, and menstrual cramps. Participants were split into groups: one camp received a myrrh supplement with a standardized extract of furanodienes, while the other received a placebo. The women who took the myrrh supplement experienced significant improvement in low back pain, as well as in pain accompanied by fevers. The men who took it experienced relief from almost all types of pain.[2]

Another study published in an Italian medical journal, *Gazetta Medica Italiana Archivio per le Scienze Mediche*, explored the effects of myrrh on tension headaches and migraines. Starting at the onset of each headache or migraine, the study participants took the myrrh supplement for seven days, and continued to do so for six months, at which time their results were assessed. The researchers found that both headaches and migraines were reduced by about two-thirds. Additionally, cytokines, which are cell-signaling compounds linked to pain, were also reduced by 40 to 60 percent, suggesting that myrrh addresses at least one causal factor for headaches and migraines.[3]

Myrrh seems to work on at least two levels: by blocking pain signals to the brain and by reducing inflammatory cytokines linked to pain and inflammation.[4] Additional animal research published in the *Journal of Ethnopharmacology* found that myrrh reduced both pain and inflammation.[5]

Myrrh has demonstrated effectiveness against migraines, which often have a wide range of possible causes, including food sensitivities, environmental factors, and hormonal changes, all of which can result in changes to the nervous system. While little research has been done on myrrh's effects on the nervous system, its ability to improve migraines suggests that it may also be helpful in the treatment of other neurological conditions, including neuropathy and trigeminal neuralgia. Research published in the journal *Evidence-Based Complementary and Alternative Medicine* also shows that myrrh essential oil helps protect the nervous system against free radicals that would otherwise cause damage.[6]

HOW TO USE

The results in the *BioMed Research International* study mentioned previously were achieved with a myrrh supplement with a standardized extract of 8 milligrams of furanodienes for women and 16 milligrams for men taken for twenty days.

In addition to standardized supplements of myrrh, I have found internal use of myrrh essential oil to be effective for the treatment of pain. Take three drops three times daily on your tongue or in an empty capsule. It's not as palatable as most people might like, so you'll probably want to take it in capsule form.

SAFETY CONSIDERATIONS

While there are many myrrh essential oil products on the market, most have been diluted with cheaper oils or contain harsh solvents used in processing, so it is important to choose an oil that has third-party laboratory testing for purity. Sadly, few companies have done this type of research, so it can be difficult to find suitable products. As most of the products are not pure enough for internal use, it is best to follow package instructions and choose a product that indicates the product is suitable for internal use and has the word *dose* on the label.

If you are applying myrrh essential oil to your skin, it is best diluted as it is quite strong. Simply dilute a couple of drops in a carrier oil like sweet almond or fractionated coconut oil. Always conduct a forty-eight-hour skin patch test of the myrrh oil diluted in the carrier of your choice prior to more extensive use. For more information on using essential oils, see page 23.

Avoid during pregnancy or while breastfeeding.

SUPER HEALTH BONUS

Myrrh may be helpful in the prevention of cancer. Preliminary research published in the scientific journal *Molecular Diversity* found that myrrh demonstrated anticancer properties against six kinds of cancer in mice (lung, cervical, breast, skin, kidney, and colon).[7] Another study in the journal *Nutrition and Metabolism* found that compounds in myrrh essential oil work by inducing cell death—a process known as apoptosis—in cancer cells.[8]

Oregano Essential Oil and Herb

(*Origanum vulgare*)

Oregano was first used by the Greeks, who believed that the goddess Aphrodite invented oregano to make the lives of humans happier. The ancient Greeks crowned newlyweds with wreaths containing oregano and placed sprigs of the herb on the graves of the deceased to help bring peace to their spirits. These ancient people also prescribed the herb regularly for the treatment of many afflictions.[1]

Perhaps the ancient Greeks were aware that, at least for those suffering from pain, oregano can indeed make people happier and ease their discomfort. And let's face it: relief from severe pain is enough to bring peace to anyone.

Oregano essential oil is one of the most versatile and potent natural medicines. Its wide-reaching and research-documented therapeutic properties make it the herb of choice for many pain conditions. Additionally, because it is a broad-spectrum antibacterial agent, it may be helpful for getting to one of the root causes of pain conditions like arthritis that have been linked to increased levels of the harmful bacteria *Prevotella copri*, which we discussed in chapter 3.

Research on carvacrol, one of oregano's active ingredients, found that it interferes with the body's pain signals between the affected part and the brain. That's great news for pain sufferers, since it can lessen the amount of discomfort we perceive and experience. In an animal study published in *Naunyn-Schmiedeberg's Archives of Pharmacology*, researchers found that carvacrol interrupted pain signals and reduced inflammation at the same time—a double-pronged approach that could have excellent effects for a wide range of pain conditions.[2]

Oregano essential oil is a potent antioxidant that prevents free radicals from wreaking havoc on the body. Free radicals are involved in the eye condition glaucoma, which causes damage to the optic nerve and can result in vision loss or blindness. Oregano essential oil, used internally, not in your eyes, may be helpful for this condition.

In a study of orofacial pain (a chronic condition involving pain of the head, neck, face, mouth, and inside of the mouth) published in *Biomedicine & Pharmacotherapy*, researchers found that carvacrol was helpful in significantly reducing the pain.[3] Research published in the journal *Frontiers in Microbiology* also showcased the effectiveness of oregano against strep infections, particularly strep throat.[4]

Due to oregano's high levels of carvacrol, as well as other possible anti-pain and anti-inflammatory compounds, oregano essential oil may be helpful in a wide variety of pain conditions, including arthritis, carpal tunnel syndrome, muscular pain, and urinary tract infections. More research into whether the anti-pain and anti-inflammatory effects of oregano make it a potential treatment for other pain disorders will likely yield interesting and beneficial results.

HOW TO USE

The best way to reap the benefits of oregano essential oil is to use it internally. You can take two to three drops of oregano essential oil in an empty capsule, three times daily, provided that you select a pure, therapeutic-grade essential oil with third-party laboratory testing to ensure purity.

SAFETY CONSIDERATIONS

Not all oregano essential oils are suitable for ingestion. Actually, most of the oregano oils on the market are not appropriate for internal use. As a result, you should use only oils that are clearly designated for internal use. This is easily identifiable on the label, which should include the word *dose* or *dosage*.

You should be aware that many of the oregano essential oil products marketed for internal use have actually been diluted with olive oil or another oil, so the dosage of two to three drops three times daily (suggested above) may not yield the desirable anti-pain and anti-inflammatory results. If you use a dropper bottle with a label that recommends squeezing the contents into your mouth, then the oil has most likely been diluted, because pure, concentrated oregano essential oil is too strong to put even a single drop in your mouth. That's why I recommend empty capsules for this purpose.

Use with caution during pregnancy. Dilute heavily for topical or oral use. Use with caution or avoid using if you have an ulcer.

SUPER HEALTH BONUS

Oregano essential oil is best known for its potent antimicrobial activity, and for good reason: carvacrol and rosmarinic acid have demonstrated antiviral, antiparasitic, and antifungal properties, all of which make it an excellent choice for dealing with infections. But perhaps the greatest health bonus is oregano's anticancer potential. While oregano hasn't been extensively studied for use against cancer, preliminary studies published in the *Journal of Medicinal Food* showed that the compound 4-terpineol found in oregano was effective at inhibiting the spread of cancer.[5] In an article in the journal *Food and Chemical Toxicology*, researchers reported that oregano targeted liver cancer cells to destroy them.[6] Considering the dreaded nature, and often deadly ramifications, of this disease, anything that offers hope and potential to people suffering from it deserves consideration, particularly when there are so few, if any, negative side effects for most people.

Peppermint Essential Oil
(*Mentha piperita*)

Although it likely began earlier, human use of peppermint has been recorded since the era of ancient Greece, where it was a staple of Greek cuisine and medicine. Also used extensively in the Middle East and by Native Americans,[1] peppermint is now grown worldwide and broadly available in food and natural medicine.

As an essential oil extracted from the plant's leaves and stems, peppermint is one of the most versatile remedies to keep in your natural anti-pain medicine cabinet. It alleviates headaches, reduces generalized muscle and joint aches and pains, and reduces inflammation. And, as an added bonus, it helps boost mood and alertness.

Peppermint, combined with black pepper, lavender, and marjoram essential oil, may also be helpful in the treatment of neck and shoulder tension and pain, according to a study published in the *Journal of Alternative and Complementary Medicine*. The researchers found that this blend of essential oils, applied in a cream base (4 percent dilution, which works out to about four drops of oil per teaspoon of cream) reduced upper shoulder tension and neck pain.[2]

Peppermint is also an excellent choice for headaches and migraines. I have recommended it for many years to clients who are chronic migraine and headache sufferers, with great results, and now research is showing that this natural prescription was well-founded. Research published in the medical journal *Frontiers in Neurology* found that applying a menthol-containing gel to the base of the skull at the onset of migraines provided significant relief for the majority of study participants.[3] Menthol is one of the main compounds naturally found in peppermint essential oil. Many of my clients, as well as many participants in my online medical aromatherapy community, have achieved similar results when they have applied peppermint essential oil to the base of the skull, temples, and other places on the head that are sore to the touch at the onset of or during a migraine.

In addition to treating headaches, migraines, and neck pain and tension, peppermint is a good choice for muscle pain and stiffness, poor circulation that causes pain or discomfort, and gastrointestinal (GI) disorders.

In an analysis of sixteen clinical studies on the effectiveness of peppermint essential oil for the treatment of irritable bowel syndrome (IBS), published in the medical journal *Phytomedicine*, researchers concluded that peppermint had statistically significant effects. It alleviated general symptoms, which include abdominal discomfort, as well as improved quality of life for people suffering from the condition.[4] It may also have an anti-inflammatory effect in the GI tract. And, as you discovered in chapter 3, reducing inflammation in the gut is a great way to improve inflammation anywhere in the body.

Another study published in the journal *Natural Products and Bioprospecting* found that peppermint and caraway essential oils were effective in the treatment of dyspepsia,[5] a condition characterized by abdominal pain and bloating.[6]

HOW TO USE

While many people drink peppermint tea in an effort to glean its anti-pain properties, this is not the most effective way to obtain the pain-alleviating properties of this analgesic herb. The concentrated extract, known as peppermint essential oil, is ideal for applying directly to painful areas of the head, neck, or body, or taking two drops on the tongue as a way to reduce pain in the GI tract. These methods are far superior to drinking the tea made from this herb.

For ease of application, I suggest that you keep a roller bottle of peppermint essential oil handy and rub it on your temples and the back of your head where the neck and head meet to help alleviate headaches.

Another great way to reap the benefits of peppermint essential oil is using it internally. You can take two drops of peppermint essential oil directly on the tongue, or two to three drops in an empty capsule, three times daily provided that you select a pure, therapeutic-grade essential oil with third-party laboratory testing to ensure purity. See the following safety considerations for more information on internal use and topical application.

SAFETY CONSIDERATIONS

Not all peppermint essential oils are suitable for ingestion. Actually, most of the peppermint essential oils on the market are not appropriate for internal use. As a result, you should use only peppermint essential oils that are clearly designated for internal use. This is easily identifiable on the label, which should include the word *dose* or *dosage*.

While peppermint essential oil can be used neat (undiluted) on the skin to help reduce pain, you may need to dilute it if you have sensitive skin. Be careful not to use too much peppermint essential oil or the fumes may cause your eyes to water. Avoid getting the oil in your eyes and be sure to wash your hands immediately after use to prevent rubbing the peppermint oil into your eyes. Also keep out of your nose and mucous membranes, and away from sensitive areas.

Use under the guidance of a qualified health professional if you're pregnant or nursing. Avoid high doses of peppermint essential oil, as pulegone, one of its naturally occurring compounds, can be toxic in high doses. See page 23 for more information on the safe use of essential oils.

SUPER HEALTH BONUS

In a study published in the journal *Phytomedicine*, scientists discovered that peppermint essential oil demonstrated high potency against the herpes virus,[7] which may make peppermint the remedy of choice for cold sores. The rosmarinic acid contained in peppermint also opens the airways and improves breathing. Additionally, while many humans love the smell of peppermint, it seems most critters can't stand the stuff. That's why it makes a great natural critter repellent. Put a few drops of peppermint oil on cotton balls around your home to ward off ants, mice, and spiders.

Thyme Essential Oil and Herb

(*Thymus vulgaris*)

Perhaps one of the most common herbs I use in my cooking, thyme adds a delicious savory taste to a wide variety of vegetable, poultry, meat, legume, and mushroom dishes. But it's not just a fragrant and versatile culinary herb; thyme is also powerfully therapeutic and can help if you're suffering from pain.

The late world-renowned botanist James Duke, PhD, author of *The Green Pharmacy*, swore by thyme's natural essential oils to effectively reduce his back spasms and pain.[1] Dr. Duke is not the only expert who has personally used and recommended thyme for pain. Many other herbalists use this powerful herbal medicine for the treatment of pain. Some recommend it in tea form (use one teaspoon of dried thyme per cup of boiled water). Others recommend soaking cloths in thyme tea to make a compress to ease aching muscles of the neck, back, and shoulders to combat tension headaches. Both options are good choices.

These visionary experts were ahead of their time in understanding the merits of thyme in the treatment of pain. A growing body of research is beginning to validate their recommendations.

The herb contains a range of medicinal compounds, including thymol, which gives thyme its highly anti-infectious properties and its signature ability to ease coughs, sore throats, and the pain of strep throat.[2] Like oregano, thyme also contains carvacrol, which may account for its impressive effects on a wide range of pain conditions. Carvacrol, which is also found in oregano, is an antinociceptive compound, which you may recall means that it blocks the perception, and possibly the transmission, of pain.

An animal study published in *Naunyn-Schmiedeberg's Archives of Pharmacology* found that not only did carvacrol interrupt the pain signals, but it also reduced inflammation at the same time—a double-pronged approach that could have excellent effects for a wide range of pain conditions.[3] While many people dismiss animal studies, and indeed, further human clinical studies are warranted, the lack of a placebo effect in studying animals makes the results of animal studies useful in better understanding natural remedies and their effectiveness against pain.

Because thyme and oregano are both excellent sources of carvacrol, it is likely that they have many similar therapeutic effects. In the same way that oregano essential oil may be helpful in the treatment of orofacial pain (a chronic condition involving pain of the head, neck, face, mouth, and inside of the mouth), thyme may be beneficial in the treatment of this type of pain. Indeed, in a study exploring the effects of carvacrol on orofacial pain, published in *Biomedicine & Pharmacotherapy*, researchers found that the active ingredient significantly reduced pain.[4]

Thyme essential oil, like oregano, may be helpful in a wide variety of pain conditions, including arthritis, carpal tunnel syndrome, muscular pain, and urinary tract infections. While scientists continue to study the effects of carvacrol, thymol, and thyme, we don't need to wait to benefit from a reduction in pain and inflammation, and improved quality of life.

HOW TO USE

The best way to reap the benefits of thyme essential oil is using it internally. You can take two to three drops of thyme essential oil in an empty capsule, three times daily, provided that you select a pure, therapeutic-grade essential oil with third-party laboratory testing to ensure purity. Thyme essential oil can be applied topically a few times daily to painful areas, but should be heavily diluted in a carrier oil since it is a strong oil that can irritate the skin.

SAFETY CONSIDERATIONS

Not all brands of thyme essential oils are suitable for ingestion. Actually, most of the thyme essential oils on the market are not appropriate for internal use. As a result, you should use only oils that are clearly designated for internal use. This is easily identifiable on the label, which should include the word *dose* or *dosage*.

Use thyme essential oil with caution during pregnancy. Dilute heavily for topical or oral use. See page 23 for more information on the safe use of essential oils.

SUPER HEALTH BONUS

As an increasing number of fungal conditions have become drug resistant, research about thyme's antifungal activity couldn't have come at a better time. Thyme has been found to be effective against *Aspergillus* spores (a common type of mold that can cause the lung condition aspergillosis)[5] and *Candida* (the culprit behind many vaginal, oral, or intestinal infections). In a study published in the *Brazilian Journal of Microbiology*, researchers found that not only was thyme effective in inhibiting growth of fungi, but it also increased the ability of the drug fluconazole to kill the disease-causing fungi.[6] Another study published in the journal *BMC Complementary and Alternative Medicine* found that thyme is even effective against drug-resistant strains of *Candida* fungi.[7]

Turmeric Essential Oil and Herb
(*Curcuma longa*)

Best known for adding a brilliant yellow color to curries and boosting brain health, turmeric is also an amazing remedy to alleviate pain and inflammation. The delicious curry spice deserves a rightful place in your daily diet and natural medicine cabinet. That's because turmeric contains multiple active ingredients that are powerful anti-inflammatories, making it effective for many types of pain disorders.

A root similar to gingerroot, turmeric contains multiple potent compounds, including the most well-known one, curcumin. Curcumin gives turmeric not only its signature yellow color but also some of the plant's anti-inflammatory properties. Curcumin appears to work by depleting the nerve endings of substance P, a pain neurotransmitter. Neurotransmitters, as the name suggests, carry signals between the brain and nerve cells. Curcumin suppresses pain through a mechanism similar to that of drugs like COX-1 and COX-2 inhibitors (without the lengthy list of harmful side effects).

In a study published in the *Journal of Biological Chemistry*, researchers found that curcumin improved the healing of tendonitis, which involves inflammation of the tendons that help maintain the body's structural integrity and mobility.[1] That's great news for anyone suffering from this condition, whether from a tennis or golf injury or another type of overuse injury involving the tendons.

In a study comparing the anti-inflammatory effects of curcumin and the drugs ibuprofen and aspirin, researchers found that curcumin was more effective than either of these drugs at reducing inflammation.[2] While the study was conducted to determine curcumin's effectiveness in the treatment of inflammation linked to cancer, its anti-inflammatory results are still relevant to sufferers of other types of pain, considering the ubiquitous nature of inflammation in most pain conditions.

Research also shows that a curcumin extract is more effective than acetaminophen or nimesulide—a potent prescription nonsteroidal anti-inflammatory drug (NSAID) that is used to alleviate pain.[3] The study reported in the *Journal of Pain Research* found that curcumin has demonstrated potent pain-relieving effects, even greater than the effects of 1,000 milligrams of acetaminophen or 100 milligrams of nimesulide. Additionally, curcumin's analgesic effects lasted longer than those of the drugs.

This new study shows that not only is curcumin an effective pain-relieving natural remedy, but it also helps prevent and heal muscle injuries and inflammation. Unlike nimesulide and acetaminophen, which have been linked to liver damage and even to deaths, curcumin has a strong safety record and has even been found to boost liver function and to protect the liver against damage.

Another exciting study published in the *Journal of the International Society of Sports Nutrition* found that curcumin could also significantly decrease muscle injury due to overactivity. Twenty healthy, active men were given either a placebo or 1 gram of curcumin twice daily. They were given the supplement or placebo starting forty-eight hours prior to a forty-five-minute downhill running race and for twenty-four hours after the athletic test to determine whether curcumin could prevent delayed-onset muscle soreness (DOMS). The researchers chose the activity of downhill running because it is known for its ability to forcibly lengthen muscles while they are in the midst of contracting, causing a stress on the body that triggers inflammation and the production of damaging free radicals, which cause muscle pain and inflammation.

Muscle damage following the period of activity was assessed using magnetic resonance imaging (MRI). Muscle damage was also assessed using blood tests and microscopic cell and tissue analyses forty-eight hours after the athletic tests. Participants also reported their levels of pain before and after the running test. The scientists found that significantly fewer people in the curcumin group showed MRI evidence of muscle injury. They also found that the curcumin group had fewer markers of muscle damage or inflammation from overexercising. This study suggests that curcumin can help prevent and heal muscle injuries, potentially even before they settle in.[4] This research may be beneficial to sufferers of fibromyalgia who experience widespread muscle pain, and who often avoid physical activity out of fear that they will experience the flare-ups linked to the disease. Curcumin may help prevent and treat the muscle inflammation linked with painful flare-ups.

There's also good news for anyone who has experienced kidney stones and wishes to prevent the painful condition from recurring. Turmeric can be helpful in maintaining a healthy urinary tract, reducing inflammation in this bodily system, and preventing kidney stones from forming. Research published in the *International Journal of Molecular Sciences* found that curcumin helps prevent kidney stones from forming in the urinary tract.[5] It appears to work by preventing them from crystallizing in the first place. Considering the excruciating nature of kidney stones, anything that helps prevent their formation will be well received by those who suffer from them.

Turmeric is helpful in the treatment of joint pain, including arthritis. In a study published in the journal *Clinical Interventions in Aging*, researchers found that turmeric was as effective as ibuprofen in the treatment of osteoarthritis of the knees.[6] The curcumin in turmeric also has a proven track record of alleviating the pain and inflammation of arthritis as well as muscle pain, making it helpful for osteoarthritis, rheumatoid arthritis, gout, and fibromyalgia.

Turmeric is also beneficial in the management and treatment of neurological pain disorders. In a study published in the *Journal of*

Ethnopharmacology, researchers found that turmeric had a neuroprotective effect,[7] meaning that it protects the nervous system from free radical or other damage that can irritate or damage the nerves and result in pain.

Multiple studies have shown that other active compounds found in turmeric, known as turmerones, may help regenerate new brain and nerve cells, which may prove useful in the treatment of nerve damage or neurological disorders. According to research published in the medical journal *Stem Cell Research & Therapy*, turmerones can cause brain stem cells to start proliferating.[8] Another study published in the same journal found that the stem cells in the nervous system, known as neural stem cells, become activated after injury or damage to the brain as a means to help regenerate the brain and nervous system and give the cells an opportunity to recover and return to normal function. The researchers found that turmerones caused an increase in the number of neurons generated by the brain or nerves. While the research was conducted for the purpose of helping Parkinson's and stroke sufferers, it may also offer hope to people who suffer from other neurological disorders or incomplete spinal cord injuries and the resulting pain that tends to accompany these injuries. It's too soon to say whether this is the case, but it's an exciting time for research, specifically for the natural remedy turmeric and its active ingredient turmerone. Considering that turmeric has a lengthy list of benefits, and few, if any, side effects, it warrants serious consideration by those suffering from neurological disorders, since they may be reluctant to wait for additional research into this application.

Turmeric can be a great option for people suffering from neuropathy or diabetic neuropathy since it works on both pain and regulation of blood sugars. Research published in the medical journal *Evidence-Based Complementary and Alternative Medicine* found that turmeric can help regulate blood sugars as well as neuropathy pain and other problems linked to diabetes.[9]

HOW TO USE

While most standardized extracts are inferior to whole herbs, this is not the case when it comes to curcumin, which is an extract from turmeric.

Both turmeric and curcumin are excellent choices for anyone seeking pain relief and a reduction in inflammation; however, curcumin typically yields superior results. Choose a standardized extract of 1,000 to 1,500 milligrams of curcumin per day. Take with meals in divided doses of 500 milligrams at a time. If you're taking curcumin supplements on their own (not with turmeric essential oil), you may want to select one that contains black pepper to improve its absorption in the body.

While it is possible to use whole-herb turmeric, it is difficult to obtain the amounts of curcumin needed to alleviate tendon, joint, nerve, or muscle pain. If you prefer to take it as food, you can take up to four tablespoons of turmeric daily mixed into water or added to juices, smoothies, soups, stews, or curries. If you're drinking it in water, you may want to add a dash of the natural sweetener stevia to make it more palatable. You'll also want to divide up that dose throughout the day, and in different dishes, since the dose is quite high and will undoubtedly add a bitter taste to your foods or beverages, which may be unappetizing.

If you're suffering from a pain disorder, however, you will likely need much higher amounts of curcumin and turmerones than diet alone can provide. Choose a standardized extract of curcumin. Follow package directions for the product you select. A typical supplementary dose is 400 milligrams per day, but discuss it with your doctor prior to use.

For conditions involving the nerves, you may also want to supplement with turmerones, which are not available in curcumin supplements and are present in only small to moderate amounts in whole-herb turmeric. The best way to obtain turmerones is by ingesting turmeric essential oil. Make sure you select a high-quality, pure, undiluted essential oil suitable for internal use. See the following safety considerations for more information about ingestion.

Ideally, you'll want to ingest both curcumin and turmerones to maximize the anti-pain benefits of this plant, particularly if you're suffering from neuropathy or another form of neurological pain. Most of the turmerone is found in the oily part of turmeric, while the curcumin is found in the ground turmeric supplements or the spice itself. You can obtain a dual-chamber supplement that contains both curcumin and turmeric essential oil (since the latter is high in turmerones). Usually these capsules have an oil-filled side and a yellow, curcumin-filled side. This combination helps you provide both compounds to the body and also increases the absorption rates of both compounds, without the need for added black pepper for absorption. I've only found one brand of this type of product, dōTERRA, which I have used with success for pain conditions.

SAFETY CONSIDERATIONS

There are few turmeric essential oils on the market. Be sure that the one you select has not been diluted with less-than-desirable oils. High-quality turmeric essential oil costs more than the cheap varieties on the market but is worth the increased price. Some cheap varieties can also contain synthetic versions of the oils, which offer no therapeutic value and may actually be harmful. But, worse than that, cheap oils are sometimes adulterated with solvents used during the extraction process or toxic pesticides used in the growing process of the herbs from which the oils are extracted. As a result, not all essential oils are suitable for ingestion. You should use only oils that are clearly designated for internal use. This is easily identifiable on the label, which should include the word *dose* or *dosage*.

Turmeric essential oil can also be applied to painful or inflamed areas. While some people can handle it neat (undiluted), it should be diluted for anyone with sensitive skin. After diluting in carrier oil, always conduct a forty-eight-hour patch test on a small, inconspicuous part of your skin to determine whether you have any sensitivity to the essential oil prior to skin application. Use turmeric essential oil with caution and with the advice of a qualified natural health practitioner during pregnancy or in the treatment of any health condition. Check with your doctor or pharmacist whether turmeric essential oil can be combined with any drugs you may be taking.

SUPER HEALTH BONUS

You may have heard about the brain- and memory-boosting benefits of turmeric and curcumin, but do you know just how quickly it starts working? Research published in the *Journal of Psychopharmacology* showed that within only one hour after taking a supplement containing curcumin, study participants had a significant improvement in memory and attention tasks compared to the placebo group.[10] Additionally, research shows that curcumin may even help protect the brain against the plaque formation found in Alzheimer's disease. It seems to work by preventing the formation of beta-amyloid plaques—which are key factors in Alzheimer's disease.[11] Even Alzheimer's patients who exhibited severe symptoms, including dementia, irritability, agitation, anxiety, and apathy, had excellent therapeutic results when taking curcumin, according to another study published in the Japanese medical journal *AYU*. In that study, participants had significant memory improvements when they supplemented with 764 milligrams of turmeric that contained 100 milligrams of curcumin every day for a year.[12]

Willow (or White Willow)

(*Salix alba* L.)

Long before aspirin ever existed, the bark from white willow trees and the herb meadowsweet were used to alleviate pain and inflammation. It was only in the last two hundred years that the pharmaceutical industry synthesized the active compounds salicin and salicylic acid, which are naturally found in these plants. The drug's common name, aspirin, reflects its original herbal heritage since the herb meadowsweet was once called spirea. Later, it was discovered that the bark of white willow trees also contained this valuable medicine. Both white willow bark and meadowsweet contain the natural, nonsynthetic version of aspirin, but because meadowsweet is harder to find and less research has been conducted on it, I'll focus my attention on white willow bark for the purpose of this book.

White willow has been used in various forms to treat rheumatoid arthritis, gout, fevers, and most types of aches and pains.[1] Research also supports the use of willow bark in the treatment of chronic low back pain, joint pain, and osteoarthritis.[2]

In a study published in the journal *Complementary Therapies in Medicine*, researchers compared the effects of white willow and the drug mefenamic acid, which is a treatment for painful menstrual periods (dysmenorrhea). They found that the women who used willow bark had superior results and a greater reduction in painful periods than those who used the drug.[3]

Research published in the medical journal *Cochrane Database of Systematic Reviews* explored studies in which white willow bark was used in the treatment of low back pain and found that the herbal remedy had better results than the placebos, demonstrating its effectiveness against the pain and inflammation linked to low back pain.[4]

Unlike aspirin—in which salicylic acid is the only therapeutic ingredient (and other synthetic ingredients, preservatives, and sometimes fillers are included)—white willow bark also contains other therapeutic ingredients, which include compounds known as polyphenols and flavonoids,[5] both of which have extensive uses due to their therapeutic properties, including against heart disease, cancer, and other conditions. Additionally, the other therapeutic compounds typically increase absorption and effectiveness, and reduce harmful side effects, when they are naturally present.

HOW TO USE

One benefit of choosing white willow bark over aspirin is that there are fewer side effects. White willow bark can be taken in tincture, capsule, or tea form. It is not necessary to take all three forms; simply use the one most readily available or most affordable to you. In my experience, tinctures tend to be the best way to take white willow bark. It is common to take 3 milliliters three times daily for pain and inflammation.[6]

If you'd prefer to drink willow bark as a tea, it is best to make a decoction, which is a boiled tea suitable for extracting the medicinal components from the roots and bark of herbs. To make a decoction, place water and one to two teaspoons of dried willow bark per cup of water in a pot. Bring to a boil, reduce the heat, and simmer for forty-five minutes. Strain the tea and drink three cups daily. You can also make the tea ahead and store in the refrigerator for up to three days.

Meadowsweet appears to be less irritating to the stomach than willow bark (though aspirin is more irritating to the gastrointestinal tract than either herb); however, it is also more difficult to find. Willow bark tends to be readily available in most health food stores.

The study published in the *Cochrane Database of Systematic Reviews* found that standardized willow bark extracts containing 120 or 240 milligrams of salicin were effective for short-term improvement of low back pain.[7]

SAFETY CONSIDERATIONS

Most of the interactions between willow bark and other drugs or other health conditions are theoretical in nature. It is often simply assumed that willow bark must have the same safety precautions as synthetic drugs containing salicylic acid (known as salicylates); however, according to some herbal experts, the salicin present in willow bark is structurally different from synthetic salicylic acid and has not been found to induce the same health problems.[8] Indeed, research indicates that fewer adverse effects are attributed to willow bark than to aspirin.[9] However, it is best to proceed with caution when using willow bark or meadowsweet. Like their synthetic drug counterparts, the herbs have blood-thinning properties and should not be taken with other blood thinners, including aspirin, or by hemophiliacs. White willow bark and meadowsweet are not recommended for use during pregnancy. Follow package instructions for these herbs. Additionally, if you have an aspirin allergy, you should avoid these herbs.

SUPER HEALTH BONUS

Because willow bark contains salicin, it acts as a natural blood thinner, making it effective for people who are suffering from atherosclerosis or heart disease. Of course, check with your doctor prior to using.

More Great Remedies
to Alleviate Pain

In addition to the essential oils, herbs, and foods we already discussed that help manage and treat a variety of pain conditions, there are many other natural remedies you can use to support your safe, drug-free healing. The panaceas in this chapter are excellent choices for many conditions, but they are more like the supporting cast than the leading ladies when it comes to their roles in alleviating pain and inflammation.

However, in some circumstances or for certain health conditions they may be among the best remedies to use. Refer to the specific pain conditions in chapter 2 for insight into the best natural options for you, especially if your budget allows for only a couple of remedies or if you want to try only a few to start with.

Be sure to give these natural medicines sufficient time to take effect, as most work on the level of healing the condition rather than just eliminating the symptoms of pain. They could take months to help heal your joints, muscles, nerves, tendons, or other tissue, so don't assume they don't work if you don't get immediate or quick pain relief.

The following remedies are in alphabetical order to help you find the ones you may wish to use. Of course, there is no need to use all of them. Even a single remedy, carefully selected and diligently used, will often yield impressive results. If you're dealing with a chronic condition, however, you may have suffered extended periods of tissue damage or injury, so you are likely better off with a few options that work against the pain and any inflammation and boost tissue healing at the same time.

ALPHA LIPOIC ACID (ALA) OR R-LIPOID ACID

One of the most potent healing nutrients is also one of the most underrated. Alpha lipoic acid (ALA), sometimes called just lipoic acid, not only functions as a super powerful antioxidant that is stronger than most but also recycles other antioxidants to keep them protecting your body against free radical damage much longer than they otherwise could. In other words, it keeps antioxidants like vitamins A, C, and E working long after they would have retired.

While not specifically a pain remedy, ALA works well to alleviate free radical damage that may be underlying some painful and inflammatory conditions, like the joint disorder arthritis or the eye disorder glaucoma. In the latter case, I've had reports that it often works quickly to alleviate eye pain. While free radical damage may be a causal factor for some painful conditions, the reality is that once a condition becomes chronic, there is most likely free radical damage playing a role, so ALA may be helpful in its treatment.

Research shows that ALA is especially good at preventing and healing inflammation and damage to the kidneys, particularly when taken along with green tea or its active ingredient EGCG.[1] A typical dose for ALA is 400 milligrams (and a typical dose for green tea extract is 300 milligrams).

Please note that sometimes other nutritional supplements are shortened to their abbreviated name "ALA," but they are different products, so be sure that the one you select is actually alpha lipoic acid or R-lipoic acid.

ASTAXANTHIN

You've probably heard of the nutrient beta carotene, which is found in many orange, red, and green fruits and vegetables like carrots, squash, and leafy greens. Beta carotene is one of a large group of nutrients known as carotenoids, which includes another nutrient called astaxanthin (pronounced as-ta-ZAN-thin). Both beta carotene and astaxanthin are antioxidants that destroy harmful free radicals before they can cause further joint and tissue damage. In their book *Astaxanthin*, researchers Bob Capelli and Gerald Cysewski demonstrate that astaxanthin is 53.7 times stronger than beta carotene in its antioxidant abilities.[2]

In a study assessing the anti-inflammatory effects of natural astaxanthin supplementation, 43 percent of participants dropped from the "high risk" classification to the "average risk" classification during the eight-week trial. The researchers examined the risk of disease linked to inflammation in the body by measuring the participants' level of C-reactive protein—a protein in the blood that tends to be elevated in response to inflammation, which we also discussed in chapter 14. While the study group was relatively small, the nutritional supplement showed great promise.[3] If this preliminary study is any indication of the possibilities for this supplement and its ability to reduce the markers of inflammation, it may be beneficial for most pain conditions.

In another small study, researchers followed twenty-one rheumatoid arthritis sufferers for eight weeks; fourteen participants were given astaxanthin while seven participants received a placebo. The participants were assessed halfway through the trial and again at the end. Researchers found that pain levels dropped by 10 percent after four weeks and by 35 percent after eight weeks, suggesting that long-term use of astaxanthin supplementation may be helpful to alleviate rheumatoid arthritis pain.[4] While more research using larger test samples definitely needs to be done, astaxanthin has been found to have benefits for so many different functions in the body—including improvement of eye health and prevention of brain diseases—that it is worth considering in the treatment of rheumatoid (and possibly other forms of) arthritis as well.

It's important to know that some forms of astaxanthin are synthetically derived from petroleum products and are not recommended; instead, choose a high-quality astaxanthin supplement derived from algae. A dose of 4 to 12 milligrams daily is suitable for the treatment of rheumatoid arthritis. Start with 4 milligrams daily, in divided doses with meals, for a month. If your pain levels have not reduced, increase to 8 milligrams daily, in divided doses with meals, for another month. If your pain levels have reduced, continue at this dosage. If after a month, they have not reduced using this dosage, astaxanthin may not be the best natural remedy for your pain disorder.

BROMELAIN

Extracted from pineapples, the enzyme bromelain normally works on digesting the natural proteins found in the fruit. (An enzyme is a specialized type of protein that acts as a catalyst for chemical processes in the body.) However, when taken on an empty stomach, bromelain works on pain and inflammation.

While some bloggers and online news sources will tell you to get your bromelain from pineapple, the reality is that fresh pineapple contains enough bromelain to digest the pineapple but is unlikely to be much help in the treatment of inflammatory conditions. Canned, heated, or cooked pineapple do not contain any bromelain as the enzymes are destroyed during the heating process. To benefit from the use of bromelain for the treatment of inflammation and the painful conditions linked to it, you'll want to use bromelain supplements. A typical dose of bromelain for conditions like muscle pain or fibromyalgia, joint pain, or tendonitis is three to five 5,000-MCU (milk clotting unit) capsules, twice daily on an empty stomach. Milk clotting units are a unit of measure for enzymatic activity.

It's important to take the supplement on an empty stomach (at least twenty minutes before meals and one hour after meals), so the enzyme can work on inflamed areas, such as sore muscles or tendons, in your body. When it is taken with meals, bromelain works on digesting the meal, not on the inflammation.

CHONDROITIN SULFATE

Chondroitin sulfate, or chondroitin, as it is frequently called, plays a critical role in the creation of cartilage. It strengthens yet provides flexibility to the connective tissue found in the joints, acts as a cushion, and helps lubricate the joints. Not only does chondroitin protect cartilage from degeneration, but it also blocks enzymes that destroy cartilage, while ensuring vital nutrients reach the cartilage for repair.

Because of its work on multiple levels to prevent further joint damage as well as to improve joint healing, chondroitin sulfate is a good choice for most arthritics but may not be necessary for those suffering from fibromyalgia.

Chondroitin is chemically similar to the blood thinner heparin, so avoid using chondroitin while taking this drug or while using other blood thinners unless you are being monitored by a doctor. You may also wish to have your doctor monitor you while taking chondroitin because it may enable you to reduce your dose of blood-thinning drugs.

Chondroitin sulfate tends to work best in conjunction with glucosamine sulfate (page 186). While there don't appear to be any toxic reactions, some people may have unwanted side effects, particularly those who are prone to severe allergic reactions; if you tend to have severe allergic reactions (the life-threatening variety), then it may be a good idea to avoid chondroitin just to be safe. If you have a shellfish allergy, avoid this supplement. Choose a sustainably sourced product because some are derived from powdered shark cartilage; others are derived from the cartilage from cows. It is not suitable for vegans; I am unaware of any vegan chondroitin products.

There are many excellent chondroitin products, including ones that combine glucosamine sulfate and chondroitin sulfate so you don't need to take as many supplements each day. Some also include MSM (page 187), so you may find that you can get all three nutrients in a single supplement. Take 1,500 milligrams of chondroitin sulfate once daily with a meal or 500 milligrams three times daily with meals.

COMFREY OIL, OINTMENT, SALVE, OR CREAM

Anyone with back pain knows how difficult it can be to get lasting relief. A long-standing Native American herbal remedy can help, according to a study published in the medical journal *Phytotherapy Research*.[5] Native Americans made an ointment or oil from an herb we know as comfrey, or *Symphytum officinale*, to treat bruises, strains, and injuries. The study found that topical applications of comfrey oil or ointment can alleviate back pain related to either muscles or joints.

The study showed that comfrey alleviates both pain and inflammation, which could explain its long and successful track record. The plant contains multiple chemical constituents that are likely responsible for its pain- and inflammation-alleviating activities. Rosmarinic acid was found to significantly reduce inflammation, while a glycopeptide found in the herb was found to inhibit four different prostaglandins that are linked with pain. Allantoin is also responsible for comfrey's pain-alleviating properties.[6]

Another study published in the *Journal of Chiropractic Medicine* found that comfrey cream was helpful in the treatment of osteoarthritis of the knees. And it doesn't just work on reducing pain, as many pharmaceutical drugs do. The comfrey cream actually speeds up the healing of tendons and cartilage. Study participants experienced a 57 percent symptom improvement after using comfrey cream for six weeks.[7]

Also known as "knitbone," comfrey has been traditionally used for bone fractures and breaks. As a result of all these applications, comfrey oil, ointment, salve, or cream may be beneficial for a wide range of pain conditions, including those involving bones, joints, muscles, or other soft tissues.

Some comfrey products contain 5 to 20 percent of the dried herb. To obtain the anti-inflammatory and analgesic actions of comfrey, choose an ointment or oil with at least 10 percent of the active ingredients from comfrey leaf (the package might say "aerial portions of the plant" or something like that). Do not exceed the manufacturer's recommended external usage. Also, choose a cream or ointment that is labeled "free of pyrrolizidine alkaloids," since they are toxic to the liver.

Because of its risk to the liver in large or long-term doses, I don't recommend using comfrey internally or using it if you have preexisting liver damage. I am not aware of any safety issue when topically using oil or ointment preparations made with comfrey, and there is lots of evidence to support their therapeutic value. Simply apply the product over the injured or sore area a few times daily until you experience improvement in your symptoms or until the wound has resolved.

ECHINACEA (*ECHINACEA ANGUSTIFOLIA, ECHINACEA PURPUREA*)

Several species of echinacea have medicinal benefits. Two of the most effective and commonly used are *Echinacea angustifolia* and *Echinacea purpurea*. Echinacea has a long history of use for reducing inflammation. Its effectiveness was demonstrated in a study published in the medical journal *Cellular Immunology*. While the study assessed the ability of echinacea to alleviate inflammation and regulate the immune system in relation to respiratory conditions, the results can be applied to other inflammatory conditions.[8]

Another study published in the online journal *PLOS One* found that echinacea was able to regulate various types of chemicals that form in the body in response to pain and inflammation, suggesting it has potential for the treatment of disorders involving these symptoms.[9]

Echinacea is also a powerful lymphatic system cleanser, which may account for at least some of its anti-inflammatory and anti-pain effects. The lymphatic system is a network of nodes, tubules, fluid, and glands that "sweeps" toxins, wastes, and by-products of inflammation out of body tissues. Echinacea helps to reduce congestion and swelling and get the lymph fluid moving, which is often an issue with pain disorders.

Research published in the *International Journal of Immunopathology and Pharmacology* found that echinacea combined with alpha lipoic acid, conjugated linoleic acid, and quercetin effectively reduced pain and other symptoms and also improved function in people suffering from carpal tunnel syndrome.[10]

Give your immune system a boost with this simple echinacea tea recipe. Stir one teaspoon of dried echinacea (flowers, leaves, stems, or seeds) or one tablespoon of fresh herb into one cup of boiled water. Let the mixture steep for ten to fifteen minutes, uncovered. You can add a touch of honey or stevia if you prefer a sweeter tea. If you're still not wild about the taste of this herbal tea, you can also add one teaspoon of dried peppermint while brewing. Drink one to three cups daily for best results.

Alternatively, take one teaspoon of echinacea tincture three times per day. Echinacea is considered an endangered plant, so be sure to do your research and choose products that have been ethically harvested.

GLUCOSAMINE SULFATE

Glucosamine sulfate is an amino sugar, a type of compound that naturally occurs in the body and is used to build tissue rather than as a source of energy like other types of sugars. It is particularly involved in maintaining healthy cartilage and bones. A glucosamine supplement is a good choice for people with arthritis or other joint disorders since they are often deficient in this compound, which naturally diminishes with age and as the body attempts to deal with arthritis.

Supplementing with this nutrient can help cartilage formation while reducing pain levels. Glucosamine has been proven in many tests to alleviate the pain of joint inflammation when taken consistently for a minimum of two weeks to two months. According to Phyllis and James Balch, authors of the classic nutrition book *Prescription for Nutritional Healing*, glucosamine has been proven in over three hundred studies to build joint cartilage.[11]

It is unlikely that you'll notice improvement within hours of taking glucosamine—that's just not how it works. To use glucosamine correctly and achieve the best results, you'll need to take it in high enough doses (1,000 to 1,500 milligrams daily) and continue taking it. Glucosamine works to halt damage to the joints and even to help strengthen cartilage, which often reduces pain, but it takes weeks or sometimes months to see results. But over time you will likely notice an improvement in pain and mobility.

Because glucosamine sulfate is usually derived from shellfish, it should be avoided if you are vegan or allergic to shellfish. If you are suffering from osteoarthritis, glucosamine works best when taken with chondroitin sulfate (page 183).

GUGGUL GUM (*COMMIPHORA MUKUL*)

Like its cousin myrrh, which you learned about in chapter 19, guggul produces a resin that is used in natural medicine, incense, and perfumery. The tree is native to Bangladesh, India, and Pakistan, and ancient texts date its medicinal uses to 600 BC.[12] Also like myrrh, guggul is an anti-inflammatory that is beneficial for osteoarthritis, rheumatoid arthritis, and other joint-related health issues and has been in use in the traditional Indian medicine known as Ayurveda.[13]

Guggul extracts contain a natural compound known as myrrhanol A that is, at least in part, responsible for guggul's potent anti-inflammatory effects.[14]

A typical dose for joint pain, including osteoarthritis and rheumatoid arthritis, is 500 milligrams of guggul (containing 3.5 percent guggulsterones), three times daily.[15]

Avoid using guggul gum during pregnancy or while breastfeeding. Little is known about its safety for use during these times. Avoid use if you are hemophiliac or have another bleeding disorder as guggul gum may slow blood clotting. Work with your physician and use with caution if you are taking any blood-thinning drugs, such as warfarin, as guggul may thin the blood. While these properties may actually be beneficial for those suffering from heart disease or arteriosclerosis, the drugs may interact with this natural medicine. If your physician approves your use of guggul gum, you may need to be monitored as it may reduce your requirements for medication. Avoid using guggul gum for at least two weeks before and after surgery.

METHYLSULFONYLMETHANE (MSM)

Methylsulfonylmethane, or MSM as it is more frequently known, is a naturally occurring sulfur compound that is found in many foods, especially dark, leafy greens. Unfortunately, most North Americans eat so poorly that there is little, if any, trace of this nutrient in the foods they consume on a regular basis. MSM is also naturally found in the body, but sometimes the amount is insufficient to overcome the inflammatory foods in our diet and our stressful lives, as well as any damage to our joints. It is therefore a good idea to supplement with this nutrient if you are suffering from joint pain or injuries. MSM helps boost joint health and healing, while alleviating pain and inflammation. MSM can also boost detoxification in the body and help restore an imbalanced immune system, making it a beneficial nutrient for any type of arthritis, including both osteoarthritis and rheumatoid arthritis, as well as fibromyalgia.

It's best to start with 1,000 milligrams total of MSM per day and build up to 2,000 milligrams daily. Eventually, you can take 2,000 milligrams daily in divided doses; for example, you can take 1,000 milligrams with breakfast and 1,000 milligrams with dinner. Because it has blood-thinning properties, avoid using MSM if you are taking pharmaceutical blood thinners, including acetaminophen. I'm not aware of any other drug interactions with MSM, but check with your doctor first.

OMEGA-3 FATTY ACIDS / DHA AND EPA

While many fats can cause inflammation and aggravate painful conditions in the body, a particular type of fat known as omega-3 fatty acids can be helpful to quell inflammation and reduce pain.

According to research published in *JAMA Ophthalmology*, eating a diet high in EPA and DHA, two types of omega-3s found in fatty fish like wild salmon, can help reduce the risk and severity of glaucoma, an eye condition associated with pain.[16] Researchers also believe that an incorrect ratio of omega-3s to omega-6s may play a causative role in glaucoma, particularly since high amounts of omega-6s without sufficient omega-3s can cause inflammation, which may aggravate the eye disease.[17]

Joel M. Kremer, MD, conducted a double-blind study, published in the medical journal *Arthritis and Rheumatism*, of forty-nine patients with rheumatoid arthritis over the course of twenty-four weeks. Dr. Kremer found that fish oils taken over the long term suppressed a

compound known as leukotriene B4, one of the main inflammatory substances linked with arthritis.[18]

As with glucosamine sulfate (page 186), many people take fish oils
and expect immediate pain relief, but the fatty acids found in fish oil
work to mend the tissues in the body, thereby improving symptoms and
overall healing over a longer period of time. While it is possible to see
immediate results, most people need to continue using fish oil supplements for a few months to obtain their full benefit. Ideally, people should
continue taking the supplements even after seeing improvement, since
they are foundational nutrients for a healthy body.

While you may be tempted to skip this supplement in favor of options
that work faster, I encourage you not to. These fats are essential to help
heal pain and inflammation at the source of the damaged tissue. Simply
going back to a deficiency state after a few months will interrupt your
healing and leave you susceptible to pain and inflammation again. Dr.
Kremer found in his study that when people with arthritis discontinue
supplementation, inflammatory leukotriene production increases again
after about one month.

Take two capsules of 1,000 milligrams of fish oils daily, for a total of
2,000 milligrams per day. Each capsule should contain at least 180 milligrams of EPA and 120 milligrams of DHA for best results. They are
best taken with food to increase absorption and to reduce the fishy
aftertaste that some people experience. If you take them with food and
still have gas and a fishy aftertaste, you may be deficient in the enzyme
lipase, which is needed to digest fats. If so, simply take a full-spectrum
digestive enzyme formula that contains lipase along with your fish oil or
DHA and EPA supplement.

Because some sources of fish have become polluted, look for a fish oil
supplement or a DHA and EPA supplement that is confirmed by third-
party laboratory results to be uncontaminated with mercury and other
pollutants. While I am not aware of any fish oil supplements being made
with genetically modified fish, as of the writing of this book genetically
modified salmon has been approved for sale in some countries, so keep
in mind that these organisms, better known as GMOs, could become a
concern in fish oil supplements in the future.

We'll discuss the role of omega-3 fatty acids and their food sources in greater detail in chapter 26.

ROSEMARY ESSENTIAL OIL (*ROSMARINUS OFFICINALIS*)

The oil extracted from the rosemary herb has anti-pain properties, is a natural nervous system relaxant, and is also helpful for the treatment of joint pain, including bursitis, osteoarthritis, rheumatoid arthritis, and gout. Additionally, it calms the nervous system, which is the route by which pain signals travel to and from the brain. Relaxing the nervous system is an important process to improve pain both in the short and long terms. Regular use of rosemary essential oil, diluted in some fractionated coconut oil or other carrier oil and applied to the affected joints, can be helpful for anyone suffering from joint pain and arthritis. Avoid during pregnancy and if you suffer from epilepsy. Follow the directions on page 23 for more information about the safe and effective use of essential oils.

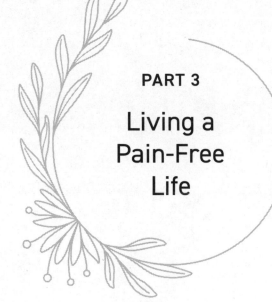

PART 3

Living a Pain-Free Life

The Pain-Erasing Diet and Lifestyle

Food is medicine. We've all heard the adage and most people know that their food choices can improve their health; however, few know just how profoundly food can affect their pain and inflammation levels. Having used my body as my personal laboratory, I was shocked at the results certain foods had on my health. I watched some foods aggravate my pain and others improve it. And I saw these results play out time after time with thousands of people I've worked with over the years.

Of course, you can reduce pain and heal using the natural remedies I've recommended in the previous chapters without changing what you eat. However, the results will be more pronounced and longer lasting when you accompany the natural medicines with dietary and lifestyle improvements. And, contrary to what you may be thinking, it's not that hard. Anyone can make some simple dietary and lifestyle changes to experience a higher quality of life.

FOODS THAT HARM, FOODS THAT HEAL

While it's equally important to eliminate the foods that act as barriers to healing, or worse, aggravate painful conditions, it's also imperative to give your body the foods it requires as building blocks for healing. It's a bit like building a home. You need to clear the site of all the debris, rocks, and brush that will get in the way of the building process, but you also need to ensure you have all the materials to build the actual house. If you try to build a house over piles of debris or without clearing the site, the house's integrity will be sacrificed. If you don't have enough building materials, you'll cut corners that will also sacrifice the integrity of your home. And that's how it is with food: you need to eliminate or remove the problem foods while also incorporating more of the healing, anti-inflammatory foods that help build healthy cells and pain-free tissues.

You won't find much discussion about junk food, fried food, or similar types of food in this book, not because they aren't harmful foods that aggravate pain and inflammation, but because it's highly likely that you already know you need to avoid these foods. Perhaps no one ever told you that you should do so to lessen your pain and inflammation, but most people realize that such foods contribute to your poor health. The reality is that these foods are just as inflammatory as they are artery clogging, cancer causing, and health debilitating. So they are best avoided as much as possible.

IT'S A FAST-FOOD WORLD

We live in a fast-paced world where everyone moves quickly to finish the next task, jet-set to the next business or holiday locale, or rise to the next opportunity. It's a race to the finish line, and as a result few people have time, or take time, for the simpler pleasures like cooking a healthy meal or savoring the foods they eat. Instead, we reach for a range of fast, convenient, and take-out foods.

This "fast-food" philosophy also reaches beyond what we eat to encompass our way of life. We want results and we want them quickly. In the same way that we want a meal in front of us in minutes, we expect quick results in all the other aspects of our lives, including the pain we experience. We expect pills to take away our suffering within minutes.

Of course, no one wants to suffer. But the fast-food mindset also absolves us from any responsibility in improving our lives. If we can take a pill to eliminate our suffering, then we don't even have to consider what factors may be contributing to the pain or what the pain is trying to tell us about the state of our bodies and health. When we quickly pop a pill that acts as a quick fix, it also becomes unnecessary for us to take measures to transform our health and set the stage for a long-term pain-free life. Of course, there are natural "pills" and remedies that can quickly and effectively alleviate pain, particularly when they are used correctly. But following my recommendations in *Pain Erasers*, including the diet and lifestyle suggestions provided here, will help ensure that you get maximum, long-lasting results. After all, isn't your goal to eliminate pain for good?

If you are willing to make the modest effort (and aren't you worth it?) required to create a pain-erasing lifestyle, the rewards are endless. By setting the stage for the best results possible through an anti-inflammatory diet and lifestyle, not only will you alleviate the inflammation linked with pain, but you'll significantly reduce the amount of pain you experience, and you'll begin to understand how simple daily choices contribute to pain or pain relief, depending on which choices you make. What's more, you'll provide your body with the nutrients it needs to heal the underlying causes of your pain—injured or damaged cells or tissues.

FOOD: THE FOUNDATION OF A PAIN-FREE LIFE

If you look around at the many food establishments or explore the way most people eat, you might be tempted to assume that we eat primarily for taste. While most people may agree with that assertion, the reality is that we eat for survival. Without food, we simply cannot live. But what happens when we eat enough food to ensure our survival but that food lacks nutrients or contains ingredients that damage the body? I believe this combination of nutrient-deficient, inflammation-causing food is playing a huge role in shaping our widespread collective pain.

While the taste of our food is important, we also need to eat food that is replete with the many macronutrients, vitamins, minerals, phytonutrients, enzymes, and other nutrients that are the building blocks of our cells so our bodies can properly maintain their strength and heal damaged areas.

For example, did you know that when you eat a meal, your digestive system (if it is working correctly) breaks down the proteins into amino acids, the complex carbohydrates into sugars, and the fats into fatty acids, and extracts the many vitamins, minerals, and other nutrients into their component parts so they can be used to make healthy cells? If any of these essential nutrients is missing, then your body simply cannot make healthy cells. And what happens when your body cannot make healthy cells? Any number of tissues become weaker or damaged, leaving you prone to injury, inflammation, and pain.

Once you understand that the body constantly removes damaged cells and attempts to replace them with new, healthy cells, you begin to realize the importance of both eating foods that contain the essential building blocks of healthy cells and maintaining a strong digestive system to break down foods into their foundational nutrients.

Before we discuss how to eat an anti-inflammatory, pain-erasing diet and improve your digestion to maximize the nutrients available to heal your joints, muscles, tendons, and other body parts that may be implicated in your pain, we'll first explore the foods that aggravate inflammation, which should be minimized in your diet for the best results.

Our standard American diet (SAD), with its high levels of sugar and high-fructose corn syrup, synthetic colors and preservatives, saturated and trans fats, genetically modified ingredients, and many other fillers and additives, is actually highly inflammatory and may be contributing to your pain.

But don't panic at the notion that you won't be able to eat most of your favorite foods, because that's simply not the case. You'll be surprised how easy it is to make simple dietary changes without losing flavor. Also, there are many ways to prepare some of your favorite dishes without using harmful or pain-aggravating ingredients, which you'll learn throughout this chapter.

The Not-So-Sweet Side of Sugar

Whenever I tell people that they need to reduce the amount of sugar in their diets, the vast majority proclaim that their diets don't include much sugar. Some people even exclaim that they don't eat many sweets, as though eating desserts was the only measure of a sugar-filled diet.

Many years ago, after my husband, Curtis, and I moved into our first home together, we did our initial grocery shopping to fill our fridge and pantry. We decided to "divide and conquer." I picked up fresh fruits and vegetables, while Curtis gathered up the pantry items and juices. He came back with freezer packages of dinner rolls and a fruit cocktail that probably didn't contain any juice at all. Suddenly, I became aware of why Curtis didn't eat desserts and why he told me that he didn't have a sweet tooth. Like most people, he believed that his diet was low in sugar when in reality many of the foods he ate contained hidden sugar. I'm happy to say that Curtis now eats an incredibly healthy diet by his own choice and that he has experienced the superior taste and health benefits of doing so. I share this story because Curtis is like so many people who think that if they don't eat desserts, candy, chocolate bars, cookies, pastries, and other sweet items, they must have a low-sugar diet, which is more myth than reality.

Thanks to the food industry, sugar is found in almost every processed, packaged, and prepared food, and even in most restaurant meals. The standard American diet, and even most healthier diets, is packed with sugar. If you compare how much sugar our ancestors ate at the beginning of the twentieth century to the amount Americans consume at the start of the twenty-first century, we actually eat a whopping *twenty-five times* more sugar. The average American now consumes approximately 152 pounds of sugar every year, which is the equivalent of fifty-two teaspoons of added sugar every day.[1] That doesn't include the sugar naturally present in fruits, vegetables, grains, and legumes.

It probably won't come as a surprise to learn that soda is among the worst culprits, since the average can of soda contains between seven and eleven teaspoons of sugar, while supersized beverages contain much more than that.

Surprising Sources of Hidden Sugar

Sugar hides in many unexpected places, so be sure to read labels to identify ingredients that end in -ose, such as glucose, maltose, fructose, high-fructose corn syrup, and so on. All of these ingredients are sugar in its myriad forms. There are also many ways that the food industry sneaks sugar into your diet,[2] even without labeling:

- The breading on most packaged and restaurant foods contains sugar.
- Sugar (in the form of corn syrup and dehydrated molasses) is often added to hamburgers sold in restaurants to reduce meat shrinkage during cooking.
- Before salmon is canned, it is often glazed with a sugar solution.
- Many meat-packers feed sugar to animals prior to slaughter to "improve" the flavor and color of cured meat.
- Some fast-food restaurants sell poultry that has been injected with a sugar or honey solution.
- Sugar is used in the processing of luncheon meats, bacon, and canned meats.
- Most bouillon cubes contain sugar (and usually MSG as well).
- Peanut butter tends to contain sugar.
- Dry cereals often contain high amounts of sugar.
- Almost half of the calories in commercial ketchup come from sugar.
- More than 90 percent of the calories found in a can of cranberry sauce come from sugar.

Sugar consumption causes rapid blood sugar fluctuations that can contribute to many pain disorders, including headaches and migraines that can be the result of high blood sugar. These headaches can occur immediately after eating sugar, or conversely, about an hour or so after eating sugary foods, as the result of excessively low blood sugar that arises at this time.

People who have insulin resistance or diabetes are especially at risk of headaches resulting from high blood sugar because insufficient insulin in response to excessive sugar consumption can keep blood sugar unnaturally high and potentially dangerous. Insulin resistance is a condition in which the body stops efficiently responding to the blood sugar–lowering effects of insulin, and is considered a precursor to diabetes.[3] Diabetes arises when a person is unable to produce sufficient insulin or use the hormone insulin effectively, which can cause blood sugar levels to rise.[4]

In addition to causing headaches and migraines, excessive sugar consumption can lead to nerve damage, which can cause a wide variety of painful conditions, including neuropathy and trigeminal neuralgia.

How to Nix Sugar Cravings for Good

Do you want your ice cream, your cake, and your candy too? What can you do when you have a sweet tooth? Well, there are many things you can do, but it's important to first understand what's happening with your blood sugar when you have cravings for sweets.

Sugar cravings typically indicate low blood sugar, which usually occurs an hour or two after eating excessive amounts of sugary foods (or skipping meals). That's because these sugary foods send your blood sugar skyrocketing to unhealthy levels, which ultimately causes your blood sugar to drop some time afterward. While the reaction of most people is to eat more sugar—and indeed, even some health professionals advise people with low blood sugar to eat chocolate bars and other sugary snacks—doing so will only cause blood sugars to plummet again later. This roller coaster can become endless.

Fortunately, it's easy to lick your sugar cravings for good with natural foods, nutrients, and food-timing tricks. Here are some of my preferred methods.

Eat Less Sugar

While it is okay to have a small amount of sugar on occasion, it is a good idea to reduce the overall amount you eat. That's something only you can do for yourself. Obviously, it will take some discipline. If you absolutely can't resist sweets, reduce the amount you normally eat. In other words, eat half of the pastry instead of the whole thing.

SNACK YOUR WAY TO BALANCED BLOOD SUGAR

Because sugar cravings often arise from low blood sugar levels, they're the body's way of letting us know that it needs more energy, or a snack or meal, to fuel our cells. But don't just choose any snack. Choose a healthy option like nuts, crudités, or fruit. Simply snacking every two to three hours on healthy snacks stabilizes blood sugar levels, stopping sugar cravings in their tracks and reducing the effects of blood sugar imbalances on pain.

CHERRY-PICK YOUR SNACKS AND SWEETS

When nothing but something sweet will satisfy your sugar cravings, eat an apple or a peach, enjoy a bowl of blueberries or other berries, or grab another favorite fruit. Fruits come with lots of minerals, vitamins, fiber, and phytonutrients that not only help slow the absorption of their natural sugars but also help heal your body and improve your overall health. There are so many delicious fruits to choose from, so keep some on hand for when you have a snack attack. Just don't overdo it, as excessive fruit consumption can also send blood sugar levels soaring. Of course, fruit is still a better option than candy, chocolate bars, pastries, or other sweets.

QUENCH CRAVINGS WITH WATER

Our body sends us messages when it needs something. It may be sending us signals that we are dehydrated, which we misinterpret as hunger pangs. I advise people to drink a large glass of pure water when they crave sweets and wait thirty minutes. Most of the time the cravings disappear. And you'll be addressing an aggravating factor for pain at the same time, since dehydration, or insufficient water intake, can worsen pain.

EMPLOY PROTEIN POWER TO ERADICATE CRAVINGS

High-protein foods break down slowly, gradually releasing energy to the body as it needs it, thereby keeping blood sugar levels stable. Most people assume that the only high-protein foods are meat or poultry, but that's not the case, and indeed many types of meat actually aggravate pain, which you'll discover momentarily. There are many excellent high-protein vegetarian foods, including lentils, chickpeas, kidney beans, pinto beans, cashews, almonds, walnuts, pecans, avocados, and quinoa, to name a few.

CHOOSE FIBER TO FIX CRAVINGS

As with high-protein foods, eating a high-fiber diet in which you eat fibrous foods every two to three hours helps stabilize blood sugar levels to prevent rapid spikes and drops, thereby reducing or eliminating cravings altogether. Fiber works because it causes the slow release of energy from the food in which it is found, resulting in ongoing, steady levels of fuel for the body without fluctuating blood sugar levels.

GET A GREAT GUT

Eat more fermented foods like sauerkraut, kimchi, and yogurt or plant-based yogurt options. Research published in the medical journal *Gut Microbes* found that probiotics in the gut can improve glucose metabolism in the body.[5] Just be sure your choices contain live cultures, which should be indicated on the package.

SPRINKLE CINNAMON ON YOUR MEALS

Research published in the journal *Lipids in Health and Disease* found that cinnamon improved all markers of the condition known as metabolic syndrome, whose symptoms include high blood sugar levels, abnormal cholesterol and triglyceride levels, and excessive abdominal fat.[6] It helps alleviate cravings while also balancing blood sugars.

SWITCH TO STEVIA

When sweetening coffee, tea, or other foods and beverages, choose stevia since it does not affect blood sugar levels. Note that stevia is not the same as Splenda, which is a brand name for a type of artificial sweetener. Stevia is an extract of the stevia plant, which is naturally sweet but does not contain sugar. We'll talk more about stevia in a bit, but first let's discuss other sugar substitutes that may actually negatively affect your health.

Other Sweeteners That Are Anything but Sweet

Before you run out to get other sweeteners to replace the sugar in your diet or assume that you're fine because your diet includes natural sweeteners, keep reading. Some of the so-called natural sugars used in processed and prepared foods, or sugar substitutes, are anything but sweet when it comes to affecting the pain and inflammation in your body.

High-Fructose Corn Syrup: The "Natural" Sweetener That Hurts

When you read the labels on candy, cereals, bread, frozen food, yogurt, baby food, granola bars, salad dressing, crackers, condiments, or other processed packaged foods, you're sure to see high-fructose corn syrup (HFCS) on the ingredients list. You might even equate commonality with safety, assuming that if high-fructose corn syrup really was damaging to your health, surely the Food and Drug Administration (FDA) would ban it, right? Wrong. Just because it has the word *corn* in it (which most people equate with a healthy vegetable) and it's found almost everywhere doesn't mean it's safe to eat.

The average American currently consumes fifty-five pounds of HFCS every year, which is a higher per capita consumption than in any other country.[7] If you're currently consuming high-fructose corn syrup (and most people are without even realizing it), it is most likely contributing to your pain and inflammation. That's because high-fructose corn syrup can perforate the gut lining, allowing partially digested food, fecal matter, and harmful bacteria to cross the intestinal wall directly into the blood.[8] The result: inflammation and an overactive immune system caused by the body's own immune system attacks on these substances, which it perceives as foreign invaders.

Additionally, sugar found in high-fructose corn syrup requires greater amounts of energy than other types of sugar in order to be absorbed by the gut. Each molecule requires two molecules of phosphorus from our body's adenosine triphosphate (ATP), which is our body's energy currency. Not only can this contribute to fatigue, but it can result in a reduction in the cellular energy available for the body's myriad other functions, including those associated with inflammation and pain, and the injured or damaged tissue typically linked to it.

Aspartame: The Sugar Substitute with a Proven Link to Pain

While foods sweetened with artificial sweeteners are billed by slick marketers as the way to have your cake and eat it too, you may want to think twice before eating these foods or adding artificial sweeteners to your foods and beverages. Makers of these chemically derived sweeteners often tout them as the healthier, low-calorie alternative to sugar, but a growing body of research indicates otherwise. They are linked to pain disorders like headaches, migraines, and joint pain.

Research presented at the Experimental Biology 2018 Conference in San Diego, California, found that artificial sweeteners can cause damage to blood vessels and impair the vascular system.[9] While that's an obvious concern for anyone (let's face it, we need blood vessels to supply nutrients and oxygen to all the organs and tissues in our body so they can work properly or heal from damage), it is of particular concern to those who are at high risk of vascular problems, such as diabetics and those who suffer from pain disorders like migraines. Sadly, diabetics are often the first people to choose artificial sweeteners and sugar-free foods that contain them.

Additionally, research also shows that aspartame in diet soda causes an imbalance in brain hormones, specifically in dopamine and serotonin.[10] These hormones help regulate pain levels as well as mood.[11]

As if that wasn't already enough reason to quit your artificial sweetener habit, aspartame has been found in animal studies, like one published in the medical journal *Nutrition Reviews*, to induce cellular damage and disrupt the integrity of the cellular membranes, potentially damaging cells and tissues, degrading their function, and leading to systemic inflammation.[12]

Additionally, multiple animal studies, including one published in the journal *Nature*, found that even small doses of aspartame can disrupt the natural bacteria found in the gut and throw off blood sugar balance in the body, both of which can further aggravate pain and inflammation.[13] A microbial imbalance may not sound like a big deal, but we're only on the cusp of discovering the many connections between our gut flora and our overall health. Scientists have already found a strong correlation between the gut and pain, inflammation, and many chronic health conditions, as we learned in chapter 3.

Lose the Sucralose and Saccharin

Does that mean you should switch to Splenda or another sugar substitute? Absolutely not. Splenda (sucralose) has been found to be a contributor to migraines in research published in *Headache: The Journal of Head and Face Pain*.[14] More research needs to be conducted on this widely used sugar substitute to determine if there are other links to pain or inflammation.

Artificial sweeteners are found in thousands of low-calorie snacks, sugar-free diet foods, and flavor syrups used in coffee and other beverages, as well as in many other foods. Yes, that includes many of the flavor additions that turn your black coffee or latte into pumpkin spice, raspberry, toffee nut, or other flavors. It's best to avoid most "diet" foods, "low-calorie" foods, or "sugar-free" foods as they are typically full of the nasty stuff. Be sure to check labels on the products to see if there are any suspect ingredients.

Stevia, the natural herbal sweetener, is the only sugar substitute that does not affect blood sugar levels, throw off gut microbial balance, damage cells or tissues, disrupt cellular membranes, or contribute to pain and inflammation. It comes in liquid or powder options. You'll use a tiny amount at a time—much less than sugar or synthetic sugar substitutes. You'll usually find a doll-size spoon in the powdered stevia bottles. One or two of these tiny spoonfuls is usually enough for adding to coffee or tea. Alternatively, you can use a few drops of the liquid stevia option. It may seem like stevia is more expensive than sugar, but a single bottle will usually last months. Of course, you should still read the labels on the stevia product you select, since stevia is sometimes diluted with less-than-healthy ingredients. You can't bake with most of the stevia products on the market without altering the liquid and dry ingredient ratios, but it is an excellent addition to beverages. I use it to sweeten freshly brewed tea and add ice for a delicious, no-sugar beverage. Stevia can, of course, be used in coffee and other drinks as well.

Refined Carbs, Bad Carbs

Sugars and artificial sweeteners aren't the only culprits when it comes to contributing to pain and inflammation. Refined carbohydrates like white rice and foods made from white flour, as well as white potatoes (which have a similar effect on the body as refined carbs), can cause rapid and far-reaching blood sugar fluctuations. The rise and fall of blood sugar contributes to low-grade inflammation anywhere in the body, as well as gut microbial changes, which, as you learned, can also cause or aggravate inflammation. Some of the offenders include pastries, doughnuts, cakes, candies, cookies, white bread, or even whole-grain or multigrain bread that is actually made from white flour with a handful of whole grains added to it.

Instead, choose whole-grain foods like brown rice, buckwheat, millet, oats, quinoa, or wild rice, along with sweet potatoes, rather than white ones. Additionally, choose 100 percent whole-grain breads to reduce the likelihood of refined flour aggravating your pain condition. It's an easy and delicious substitution once you get used to it.

Good Fat, Bad Fat

You'll also want to become more aware of the types of fats you're eating and how they may be contributing to your pain levels. There are many different types of fat, but it isn't necessary to learn about all the different ones to start experiencing a reduction in pain.

You may have heard of omega-3 and omega-6 fatty acids, which we briefly discussed in the previous chapters. Basically, you'll want to reduce your consumption of omega-6 fatty acids while also increasing your omega-3s.

It's easy to eat excessive amounts of omega-6 fatty acids without realizing it. Although they are actually healthy fats when consumed in a 1:1 or even 2:1 ratio of omega-6s to omega-3s, most people eat them in a 20:1 ratio and some people get a 40:1 ratio. The excess worsens and even causes inflammation in the body, contributing to pain.

While omega-6 fatty acids are found in most foods, they are found in the highest concentrations in corn, sunflower, and safflower oils, as well as in the meat of animals that eat a diet high in these fats. Most prepared, processed, and packaged foods contain these oils. Even most "vegetable oil" people use for cooking and baking contains these fats.

The standard American diet, most ketogenic diets, the Atkins diet and other high-protein diets, and most other fad diets contain excessive amounts of omega-6 fatty acids. With the exception of the standard American diet, most people think these diets are healthy, but they can actually be contributing to the aggravation of many pain disorders thanks to their unhealthy fat ratios.

In addition to directly contributing to inflammation in the body, many of these diets are high in animal protein and, therefore, saturated fat, and both of these also contribute to inflammation and an imbalance in gut microbes when they are eaten in high amounts, which is the case in the standard American diet.

Of course, it should come as no surprise that fried food is also a serious threat to those suffering with pain disorders. Not only are most oils used in the frying process high in omega-6 fatty acids, but they are usually heated and reheated to temperatures high above their smoke point. The smoke point is the lowest temperature at which an oil will begin to smoke. The smoking of oil is a clear sign that the oil will cause inflammation in the body, due to the change in chemical makeup it undergoes when it smokes. If you're cooking with oil and it begins to smoke, it is best to throw it out (not into the water system, though, as doing so contributes to ecological damage) and start again with fresh oil. Once you get used to this, you'll be able to easily tell when an oil is getting too hot and will soon start to smoke. You'll also be able to tell the difference between the evaporation of water in foods in the form of steam, and smoke. Steaming is fine; smoking is not.

Most people don't realize that the many cooking and baking oils they use have already surpassed their smoke point by the time the oils, or the foods made with them, reach the grocery store shelves. The oils are heated to excessively high temperatures during the manufacturing processes. If you've ever seen the term *cold-pressed* on bottles of oil found in health food stores, that will give you some insight into the superiority of these oils. Cold-pressed oils are extracted without heat, which helps to ensure the integrity of the fatty acids they contain. Of course, if they are corn, vegetable, sunflower, or safflower oils, they will still contain high amounts of omega 6-fatty acids, but they will be better choices than oils that have been excessively heated prior to arriving in your kitchen.

It's also wise to reduce your meat consumption. Not only are diets high in animal protein full of saturated fats that can aggravate inflammation, but animal proteins release acidic by-products that can build up in the tissues and worsen pain and inflammation. This is especially true for anyone suffering from a joint condition like gout, arthritis, or bursitis. It's not necessary to eliminate meat completely, although, of course, you can if you want to. But I recommend significantly cutting back. And when you choose to eat meat, choose fish or lean poultry over red meat or processed meats.

Additionally, it is best to avoid peanuts, peanut oil, and foods cooked in peanut oil because they tend to contain molds known as aflatoxins that can severely aggravate joints and tissues, causing pain and inflammation.

Trans fats are harmful to every cell in your body, but especially your brain, where pain signals are regulated. These fats do not occur naturally and are made in laboratories and manufacturing plants where oils are heavily processed. This processing involves adding hydrogen atoms to a fat to saturate the fat molecules, thereby turning unsaturated oil into saturated oil. The result is a hydrogenated fat, or trans fat, which our bodies were never intended to ingest or digest. Hydrogenated fats are an industrial creation designed to extend the life of fats without regard for the effect on pain, inflammation, or human health. Even a few generations ago, our ancestors were never exposed to these toxic ingredients that have no place in our diet.

And the omnipresence of trans fats spells more bad news for people who are deficient in omega-3 fatty acids, since these people will absorb up to twice as many trans fats when eating them, making these people even more vulnerable to their inflammatory effects.

If you think you're not eating trans fats, here's just a sampling of the places they lurk: margarine, crackers, cookies, pies, vegetable shortening, snack foods, prepared and packaged salad dressings, doughnuts, and French fries. The list also includes most restaurant foods. For many years, margarine has been billed as a healthy alternative to butter, but many brands of margarine contain trans fats or rancid fats that are best left behind. Margarine is cheap to make, so many manufacturers have profited from the misleading marketing.

And if you think, "Well, I read the packages of the foods I eat and they always say '0 grams trans fats,' so this doesn't apply to me," you're wrong. That's because small amounts of trans fats are allowable in most foods, provided they are less than a gram. So even when the label says "0 grams trans fats," the food may still contain trans fats—less than other products, but no amount of these toxic fats is safe. And when you add up these hidden trans fats, they still spell damage to your cells and tissues, which ultimately means more pain.

Getting More Good Fats

Essential fatty acids are critical to balancing inflammation and pain in the body because they're the precursors of inflammation-regulating chemical messengers known as prostaglandins. Prostaglandins are made from omega-3 and omega-6 fatty acids. Both types of essential fatty acids are required, but the ratio is what matters most. The vast majority of the population is deficient in omega-3 fatty acids, which can cause inflammation to go unchecked in the body.

Omega-3 fatty acids are primarily found in the oils of cold-water fish, such as salmon, mackerel, herring, sardines, and anchovies, as well as nuts and seeds like flax, hemp, and walnut. Add flax oil or flaxseeds to your salad dressings, organic popcorn, oatmeal, smoothies, or other foods on a daily basis for best results. If you suffer from gout, you'll want to read more on page 48 before adding foods like mackerel, herring, sardines, or anchovies to your diet.

Thanks to low-fat diet fads, many people incorrectly believe that fat is not essential to the health of our bodies. But dietary fats are broken down into components known as fatty acids, the building blocks of fatty components of the body, including the nerves, which transmit pain in the body. Ensuring a healthy nervous system helps reduce pain.

By supplementing with fish, flax, walnut, or pumpkin seed oil, you can quickly restore a healthy ratio of omega-3 to omega-6 fatty acids in your body. Fish oils are among the best supplements for reducing inflammation thanks to two active essential fatty acids known as eicosapentaenoic acid (EPA) and docosahexaenoic acid (DHA), both of which have been found in numerous studies to be helpful for many inflammatory conditions. These two types of omega-3s convert in the body into hormonelike substances that decrease inflammation. According to some estimates, fish oil acts directly on the immune system by suppressing the release of cytokines, compounds that are known to destroy tissues and tend to be a concern in pain disorders.

If you're fighting inflammation, it's wise to eat fish daily or supplement with fish oil capsules daily. It takes more fish oil to lessen inflammatory conditions than to prevent them or to prevent further tissue damage. Once your symptoms level off, you may be able to reduce your dosage of fish oils or obtain your fish oils from eating fatty fish several times a week. I prefer a supplement combination of DHA and EPA, since both of these fats are needed to reduce inflammation in the body. People who are deficient in omega-3 fatty acids absorb twice as many fatty acids once they start supplementing with them as people who already have sufficient amounts. In my experience, most people with pain disorders lack sufficient omega-3 fatty acids in their diets and will find that they readily absorb these important nutrients when they make an effort to obtain them in their diets.

Food Additives

Carbs and fats aren't the only dietary factors you'll want to consider—synthetic food additives used in the manufacture of prepared, packaged, and processed food can also aggravate pain and inflammation. While any food additive may be a concern, and indeed, few additives have been tested for their inflammatory effects, one in particular stands out as necessary to avoid if you suffer from pain and inflammation.

Carrageenan: The Hidden Food Ingredient That Is Linked to Pain and Inflammation

There's a questionable additive so ubiquitous in the food industry that even many foods that have been "certified organic" contain it: carrageenan, which acts as a thickener or emulsifier for many prepared foods. Many people who are familiar with carrageenan believe it is a harmless extract from a seaweed known as Irish moss. But researchers actually use carrageenan to induce pain and inflammation in animal studies when testing the effects of analgesic drugs.

Dr. Joanne Tobacman, one of the principal scientists studying the effects of carrageenan consumption, has conducted multiple studies about this harmful food additive, including one that was published in the *Journal of Diabetes Research*. After only six days, animals fed carrageenan developed glucose intolerance, which is an umbrella term used to describe impaired metabolism involving excessively high blood sugar levels. Dr. Tobacman found that the food additive caused blood sugar levels to skyrocket, indicating that it may lead to the development of diabetes. She states that the carrageenan used in animals' diets so commonly causes diabetes that the additive could be used for mouse models of the study of diabetes.[15]

Dr. Tobacman also found that carrageenan causes intestinal and systemic inflammation in animal studies.[16] Her research also suggests that the amount of carrageenan found in most peoples' diets is sufficient to cause inflammation.

Carrageenan is found in many common foods, including ice cream, cream, butter, soy milk, almond milk, rice milk, cottage cheese, sour cream, yogurt, coffee creamers, vegan cheese alternatives, eggnog, deli meats, grocery store rotisserie chickens, juices, puddings, pizzas, chocolate bars, and coffee beverages. Additionally, aloe vera gel and some supplements, particularly gel caps, commonly contain carrageenan.

For more information on foods that contain carrageenan, check out the website of the Cornucopia Institute, which has compiled a comprehensive list of organic foods that contain carrageenan.[17] It's important to keep a list like this one handy while grocery shopping since the ingredient is legally allowed in foods bearing the label "organic" or "certified organic."

※

Once you've removed many of the pain- and inflammation-aggravating foods from your diet, you'll also want to start adding foods that can help reverse pain and inflammation. Fortunately, there are many excellent options.

SOME OF THE BEST FOODS THAT FIGHT INFLAMMATION AND PAIN

Some of the best healing remedies to overcome inflammation also taste fabulous—I can't say that about any prescription medications I've come across. Plus, foods won't cause the nasty side effects common to most pain medications. You learned earlier in this book about foods like chilies, ginger, and turmeric in their concentrated medicinal forms, but they also warrant a mention here because they are among the best foods to fight pain. You also learned that the inflammation-causing foods mentioned earlier in this chapter can be replaced with better options, which I hope you'll add to your diet. In addition to eating more of these foods, try eating the following foods to fight inflammation and pain.

Blackberries

Often overlooked, blackberries offer impressive health benefits in addition to their delicious taste. According to research published in the *International Journal of Molecular Sciences*, blackberries and their components, known as anthocyanins, help prevent inflammatory disorders.[18]

Blueberries

Blueberries are also excellent anti-inflammatory foods. They regulate the amounts of compounds called heat-shock proteins in the brain, thereby reducing inflammation linked to neurodegenerative disorders, according to a study published in the journal *Neurobiology of Aging.*[19]

Cherries

In a study published in the Spanish medical journal *Nutrición Hospitalaria*, researchers found that eating tart cherries was effective in the treatment of exercise-induced muscle damage and the inflammation accompanying it.[20]

Dark Green Veggies

Veggies such as kale and spinach contain high amounts of alkaline minerals like calcium and magnesium. Both minerals help balance body chemistry to alleviate inflammation.

Fish

Fish, and the omega-3-rich oil it contains, acts directly on the immune system by suppressing the release of inflammation-causing cytokines—an underlying factor for most pain conditions.

Flaxseeds and Flax Oil

Flaxseeds are also high in omega-3 fatty acids that reduce inflammatory substances. You can add ground flaxseeds to smoothies, top pancakes or French toast with them, or add them to many other foods. While they can be added to baked goods, they are best left unheated.

Olive Oil

The inclusion of olive oil is one of the reasons for the Mediterranean diet's many health benefits. That's because olive oil is rich in oleic acid, an omega-9 fatty acid that has anti-inflammatory properties. Research published in the journal *Nutrients* found that olive oil consumption reduced the markers of inflammation.[21] Other research published in the *International Journal of Molecular Science* found that olive oil quashes pain similarly to NSAIDs.[22] A powerful compound known as oleocanthal found in extra-virgin olive oil inhibits inflammatory enzymes the same way drugs like ibuprofen do. You can drizzle olive oil over your salads, roasted vegetables, or baked sweet potato. Just be sure not to heat it beyond its smoke point because it will no longer offer therapeutic benefits and may actually increase inflammation at that point.

Pomegranates

Pomegranates help alleviate joint pain and inflammation, according to research conducted by the National Institutes of Health. The researchers found that pomegranate fruit extract had a beneficial effect on markers of inflammation and cartilage degradation in arthritic joints, known as matrix metalloproteinases (MMPs).[23]

Pumpkin Seeds

Thanks to their rich omega-3 content, pumpkin seeds may be effective in the treatment of pain disorders, particularly those in which inflammation is a concern. A classic study published in the journal *Pharmacological Research* found that pumpkin seed oil yielded anti-inflammatory results similar to those of the pain drug indomethacin—without the side effects.[24]

Strawberries

Strawberries aren't just delicious; they also offer pain and inflammation relief. In a study published in the scientific journal *Nutrients*, researchers found that eating strawberries regularly helped alleviate the pain and inflammation of osteoarthritis in the knees.[25]

Walnuts

Like flax and pumpkin seeds, raw, unsalted walnuts contain plentiful amounts of omega-3 fatty acids, which decrease pain and inflammation. If you're like many people, you may be thinking that you don't like walnuts, but I encourage you to try the fresh ones kept in the refrigerator section of your local health food store, as they have a rich, buttery taste, without the bitterness found in the rancid walnuts in many grocery stores.

ADOPTING A PAIN-ALLEVIATING LIFESTYLE

By now, you're aware of the necessary dietary changes to make if you want to experience less pain, but it's equally important to recognize that pent-up emotions or trauma can be a causal factor for your pain. Additionally, high levels of stress can worsen pain and make it more difficult for your body to heal any injuries or damaged tissue. So it's important to find ways to express unresolved emotions, address high stress levels or at least better support your body's ability to deal with stress, and, of course, get sufficient exercise to support healing without aggravating pain and injuries.

Chronic pain and emotions are heavily intertwined. It's difficult to separate emotional and physical pain because they are so interwoven. I have observed this fact over and over in my practice with thousands of patients. Most chronic pain sufferers are also suffering emotionally, whether it be from the loss of loved ones; unrequited love; emotional, physical, or sexual abuse; trauma linked to injuries or accidents; or events a person has witnessed.

The resulting anxiety or depression often initiates or aggravates chronic pain. Many studies show the connection between what people often refer to as "negative emotions" and chronic pain. Some experts claim that people with depression are three times as likely to suffer from chronic pain.[26]

According to a study published in the *Journal of Clinical Psychology*, "Psychological research demonstrates that greater pain is related to emotional stress and limited emotional awareness, expression, and processing. Social research shows the potential importance of emotional communication, empathy, attachment, and rejection."[27]

While most emotions, including the so-called negative ones, are normal and most of us experience anger, sadness, grief, and other feelings, we need to find a healthy release to prevent them from bottling up inside our bodies. There are many ways to alleviate the stress and difficult emotions that may be underlying factors for your pain.

It's important to release any pent-up emotional pain wherever possible, take measures to reduce stresses, and support your body's ability to cope with any remaining stresses or the impact of the stress.

Take Up a Creative Pursuit to Alleviate Pain

Sing, dance, paint, draw, write, or find another creative outlet for your feelings. Many people find that they had an interest in creative pursuits but gave them up when the realities of making a living hit. But getting back to these means of creative expression can act as a release valve for pent-up emotions. Even if you've never tried such activities, doing so is worth considering.

Journaling how you're feeling each day can help you access emotions that are stored in your body, providing an outlet for their expression. It may feel difficult to get started, but once you do, you'll quickly find that the words flow.

Spend Some Time in Nature

Have you had your daily dose of trees, flowers, and shrubs? I don't mean in the form of herbal medicine, although by now you're well aware of how plant medicine can help with your pain. I'm referring to spending time communing with nature. We all know that spending time in nature just feels great, but even the research supports it. According to a study published in the medical journal *Proceedings of the National Academy of Sciences of the United States of America*, there are more reasons than ever to get outdoors and spend time in nature: the experience transforms your brain and reduces your risk of mental illness.[28]

Scientists at Stanford University in Stanford, California; the Royal Swedish Academy of Sciences in Stockholm, Sweden; and the Laureate Institute for Brain Research at the School of Community Medicine in Tulsa, Oklahoma, set out to understand why the increasing trend of living in cities is linked to an increased risk of mental illnesses like anxiety or depression. To do so, they compared brain activity of individuals who took walks in urban settings to that of those who walked in natural settings. Additionally, they assessed the individuals' tendency to engage in rumination—a repetitive form of thought focused on negative aspects of the self and a known risk factor for mental illness.

They found that the study participants who took ninety-minute walks through nature reported lower levels of rumination and showed reduced brain activity in an area of the brain known as the subgenual prefrontal cortex (sgPFC)—a region in which high activity has been linked to mental illness. The participants who took the ninety-minute walks in urban settings experienced no difference in rumination or brain activity. The researchers concluded that "these results suggest that accessible natural areas may be vital for mental health in our rapidly urbanizing world."

In a British study published in the journal *Landscape and Urban Planning*, researchers found that people who live in more densely forested areas are less likely to be taking antidepressant medications, which are in common use among pain sufferers. These scientists explored the association between urban green spaces and mental well-being and found that an increased tree density in cities significantly reduces the rate of antidepressant prescription and use. After making adjustments for other possible factors, the researchers found that every additional tree per kilometer of street resulted in 1.18 fewer antidepressant prescriptions. In this study, researchers concluded that increasing the number of trees may reduce the incidence of depression.[29] Now, that's a prescription I can get on board with.

Talk It Out with a Loved One

Most of us feel a sense of relief when we talk about a difficult experience with a trustworthy loved one. Just expressing the emotions and knowing someone else cares can make us feel like we've had a heavy weight lifted off our shoulders. Unburdening ourselves of pent-up feelings and emotions can also help alleviate physical pain. Of course, it's not always possible to talk to loved ones. But even if they've passed away, it can be helpful to have an imagined conversation with them about any issues we may be facing.

Alternatively, you may find it helpful to talk to a counselor or psychologist who can help you work through any traumas or other stresses that may be underlying your physical pain. There are many excellent options, so if one doesn't work out for you, try another one. There are also many affordable options in your community, so it's a good idea to reach out to help unburden yourself from any emotional pain that may be underlying your physical pain.

Eliminating the Source of the Stress

Find the source of the emotional stress you face. Of course, experiencing physical pain plays a role in aggravating stress levels. But ask yourself where in your life you may have experienced emotional trauma or pain. Then determine whether there is a current source of stress that may still be affecting you, and wherever possible, eliminate the source of the stress. Of course, it may not always be possible, but by eliminating any stresses you can from your life, you'll be taking strides toward a pain-free life.

Say No to Situations or People Who Stress You Out

We all have situations or people in our lives who sap our energy. While it may not be possible to eliminate all of these energy thieves, it can be surprising how many you can actually live without. Make a list of the situations you dread or the people in your life who sap your strength and create stress in your life. Make an honest assessment of what or who you could really do without or who you could see less frequently. Life is too short to spend it doing things you can't stand. Additionally, it's important to surround yourself with supportive people who bring out the best possible you, not stress you out.

Meditate Your Way to Pain-Free Peace

While most people associate meditation with religion, this simple and powerful practice transcends religious beliefs. Meditation is like a short vacation away from the stresses of everyday life to allow you to center your mind and create a peaceful feeling. And a growing body of research shows that meditation benefits your health in many ways, including improving mood, improving pain threshold, activating the immune system, decreasing stress hormones, and helping reverse the effects of chronic stress. Daily practice offers the greatest benefits. Over time it becomes easier. By meditating on a regular basis, you can train your mind to relax and release stress.

There are several ways to meditate: breathing meditation, walking meditation, sitting meditation, mindfulness meditation, guided meditation, and visualization. Choose the type that has the most appeal for you and best fits with your lifestyle and abilities. Breathing meditation is one of the easiest and most convenient forms of meditation. It can be done anywhere at almost any time, even if you have only a few minutes. It requires no special equipment other than your lungs. You can do a breathing meditation while you are waiting in a doctor's office, standing in a grocery store line, or sitting at your desk. You can use a regular reminder throughout the day to help you remember to breathe deeply. You could choose to take deep breaths on commercial breaks while watching television or at red lights while you are traveling.

Make time for meditation, even if it is on the bus ride home from work or while you are sitting in your office, but try to practice it daily. The potential rewards and freedom from pain are worth far more than the time and effort it takes to meditate.

Take a Nutritional Approach to Reduce Stress

We may unknowingly be doing things that stress our bodies out, which can initiate or worsen anxiety and depression. It's important to support our bodies nutritionally to reduce stress. Here are some of the best ways to do so.

Don't Skip Meals

Low blood sugar is a serious stress to the body that results in a cascade of stress hormones. While an occasional boost of these hormones might be fine, over time this chronic stressor can actually cause massive swings in blood sugar levels that can worsen feelings of sadness or depression, aggravate tissue damage, and worsen pain.

Eat a High-Fiber Diet

You may be wondering how fiber can help alleviate stress. In addition to eating every few hours to ensure that your body has a constant supply of energy for healing, eating a diet that is high in fiber can ensure the slow release of blood sugar and sustain it over hours, which means an end to fluctuating blood sugar levels and their ability to aggravate pain and worsen moods. To boost your fiber intake, sprinkle flaxseeds or hemp-seeds on your cereal, add a half cup of beans to your next soup or salad, and thicken your next smoothie with a tablespoon of chia seeds (drink it up quickly or it will turn to pudding!).

Take a Vitamin B Complex and Vitamin C Supplement

B complex vitamins and vitamin C are not stored in the body, so it is imperative to obtain adequate amounts from food and supplements every day. Without adequate B complex vitamins, we become susceptible to stress, depression, and irritability. Our bodies deplete high amounts of vitamin C when we're stressed, yet this essential nutrient is needed to fight free radicals that could otherwise damage inflamed or injured and painful areas. B vitamins are largely found in brown rice, root vegetables, citrus fruit, strawberries, cantaloupe, kale, and green vegetables. In addition to eating these foods, take a 50-milligram B complex supplement on a daily basis (some of these vitamins are measured in micrograms [mgc], so you'll take 50 micrograms in those cases). Vitamin C is found in oranges, lemons, grapefruit, limes, pomegranates, strawberries, black currants, spinach, beet greens, tomatoes, sprouts, and red peppers. Most nutrition experts recommend a 500-milligram supplement of ascorbic acid, calcium ascorbate, or magnesium ascorbate, all of which are natural forms of vitamin C, as a daily minimum.

While these simple dietary and lifestyle changes may not alleviate all your stress, they may help make it more manageable and give your body the tools it needs to help you better cope with life's challenges.

Move Your Body to Alleviate Emotional and Physical Pain

Anyone who has experienced the health and emotional benefits of taking a brisk walk, going for a long bike ride, or working out at a favorite health club or, better yet, in nature, knows that exercise has physical and emotional benefits. Our bodies were meant for movement, and while it is not always possible if the root cause of our pain is an injury that impairs mobility, in most cases exercise, even gentle forms, can be beneficial.

Researchers at Australia's University of Sydney and Macquarie University, as well as the Federal University of Minas Gerais in Brazil, have determined that exercise is one of the most powerful tools to prevent low back pain. Published in the American Medical Association's journal *JAMA Internal Medicine*, their research reveals that strategies such as education, sick leave, back belts, or protective shoe insoles alone offer minimal improvement of back pain; however, exercise alone or in combination with back health education offers the best results in preventing low back pain.[30]

The study found evidence that exercise alone contributed to a 35 percent risk reduction for a low back pain episode and a 78 percent risk reduction for sick leave. The combination of exercise and education contributed to a 45 percent risk reduction for a low back pain episode. Interestingly, the positive effect decreased (exercise and education) or disappeared (exercise alone) in the longer term, which was defined as greater than one year. The researchers determined that for exercise to remain protective against future low back pain, ongoing exercise is required and prevention programs focusing on long-term behavior change in exercise habits are important.

While exercise can take the form of walking, jogging, hiking, biking, and other vigorous forms of activity, it does not have to involve extended periods of high-impact, aerobic activities. Your body will thank you if you incorporate low-impact exercise that supports biomechanically correct movement and stretching, as well as proper breathing. Yoga, for example, is an effective means to prevent back pain and can be practiced in the privacy of your own home or in a social setting if you prefer to exercise in groups.

Smell Your Way to Stress Relief

There are many great essential oils that can help alleviate stress, but some of the best ones are black spruce, clary sage, frankincense, geranium, ginger, lavender, lemon, pine, rosemary, wild orange, and ylang-ylang.

Black Spruce

The delightful natural forest scent of black spruce is believed to help regulate stress hormones in the body, thereby helping us better cope with the daily stresses of life.

Clary Sage

Clary sage essential oil has been shown in an animal study published in the *Journal of Ethnopharmacology* to balance the brain hormones linked to depression (which, as you learned in chapter 1, is a common experience for pain sufferers), making it a novel potential treatment for those suffering from this mental illness.[31]

Frankincense

In a study published in the *Journal of Psychopharmacology*, a natural compound found in frankincense was found to have antidepressant qualities. The compound, known as incensole acetate (IA), was found to regulate hormones.[32] The researchers concluded that frankincense has potential as a novel treatment for depression. When a pure enough quality of essential oil is used, frankincense can be used internally by adding a couple of drops to an empty capsule and taking it three times daily. Of course, it is best to follow the safety considerations found on page 25 when using suitable essential oils internally.

Geranium

In a study published in *Complementary Therapies in Clinical Practice*, researchers assessed the effects of geranium essential oil on anxiety levels and found that it was significantly more effective than a placebo at reducing anxiety.[33]

Ginger

The essential oil of gingerroot helps modulate stress hormones while also helping alleviate pain and inflammation in the body. It is particularly effective when used internally for these purposes. Of course, it is best to follow the safety considerations found on page 25 when using suitable essential oils internally.

Lavender

Researchers found that lavender was about as effective as a common drug used in the treatment of depression.[34] In another study published in the medical journal *Frontiers in Pharmacology*, researchers attribute the antidepressant effects of lavender essential oil (and its naturally present compound linalool) to its ability to help regulate the brain messenger known as serotonin. Serotonin, one of the body's feel-good chemical compounds, is imbalanced in people suffering from depression.[35]

Lemon

The fresh, bright scent of lemon is valuable for more than just cleaning your home—it can actually help ward off depression. According to an animal study in the journal *Behavioural Brain Research*, scientists found that lemon was effective in the treatment of depression.[36]

Pine

The essential oil of pine trees has been used for many years to help alleviate stress, plus it conjures images of a pleasant forest walk. It is believed to work by quelling excess amounts of stress hormones.

Rosemary

Rosemary has been found to have a potent antidepressant effect on animals studied. A study published in the *Journal of Ethnopharmacology* found that the long-term traditional use of rosemary as a treatment for depression was justified. Researchers found that the extract reversed depression in animals about as well as the drug fluoxetine;[37] it is likely that the essential oil would have similar effects.

Wild Orange

Wild orange or sweet orange essential oil is an uplifting oil that boosts mood and is a great all-natural anxiety remedy. In a study published in the scientific journal *Physiology & Behavior*, researchers found that people who inhaled orange oil prior to dental treatments had lower levels of anxiety, an increase in calmness, and a better mood than those who did not inhale it.[38]

Ylang-Ylang

Preliminary research published in the *Journal of Ethnopharmacology* found that ylang-ylang not only balances brain hormones linked to anxiety but also helps reduce stress hormones.[39]

You can diffuse one or more of the above essential oils in an aromatherapy diffuser for at least twenty minutes to reap their antidepressant effects, or you can simply inhale the oil several times throughout the day for at least a few minutes each time. Alternatively, add a few drops of the oil to a cloth, and carry the cloth with you and sniff it throughout the day. Or place the cloth on your pillow to breathe in the scent during the night while you sleep.

You can also dilute one or more of the essential oils in a carrier oil like fractionated coconut oil or sweet almond oil and apply to the wrists, back of neck, chest, or other areas to help reduce stress. Oils such as black spruce, clary sage, geranium, pine, and ylang-ylang should not be used internally. See page 23 for more information about the safe and effective use of essential oils.

Regardless of the ways you choose to release pent-up emotions, reduce stress, and help your body cope with stress, doing so is likely to make you feel better emotionally while also reducing physical pain.

ACKNOWLEDGMENTS

To Curtis, for always believing in me, for treating me like a queen, and for picking up the slack around our home and acreage as I wrote this book, as well as the many ways you've helped me to deal with the pain I experienced over many years.

To my amazing agent and dear friend, Claire Gerus, for always believing in me and for your constant support for this project and my work. Your commitment to excellence shows in everything you do, including this project.

To Glenn Yeffeth, Vy Tran, and all of the exceptionally professional team at BenBella, for your belief in this project and your excellent work to turn this into the lovely book it has become, and one that will help many people.

To Dr. Robert Laquerre at Alta Vista Chiropractic in Ottawa, Ontario, Canada, for getting to the root problems behind the pain I experienced and giving me hope again.

To my sister, Bobbi-Jo Meyer, and mom, Deborah Schoffro, for all your support and encouragement with my work in essential oils.

To my dear old dad, Michael Schoffro, for everything you do and for being such a great dad.

To Jane Mullin Schweitzer, for all your support for my work with essential oils.

To the wonderful and unmatched team of baristas at the Kemptville Starbucks, for cheering me on, helping to keep my mind sharp with your witticisms, providing me with fuel, and for your friendship and support as I became your self-appointed writer-in-residence.

To my team of amazing women and men who have chosen to share their journey with essential oils with me.

NOTES

Introduction

1. James Dahlhamer et al., "Prevalence of chronic pain and high-impact chronic pain among adults—United States, 2016," *Morbidity and Mortality Weekly Report*, September 14, 2018; 67(36): 1001–6, www.cdc.gov/mmwr/volumes/67/wr/mm6736a2.htm, accessed March 2, 2020.

Chapter 1

1. "What causes chronic pain?" www.webmd.com/pain-management/guide/cause-chronic-pain, accessed March 1, 2020.
2. Ibid.
3. Personal interview with Robert Laquerre, January 2013.
4. D. C. Kerrigan et al., "Knee osteoarthritis and high-heeled shoes," *Lancet*, May 9, 1998; 351(9113): 1399–401, https://pubmed.ncbi.nlm.nih.gov/9593411/, accessed January 3, 2020.
5. Adam Felman, "What is pain, and how do you treat it?" www.medicalnewstoday.com/articles/145750, accessed January 31, 2020.
6. Peter C. Gøtzsche, "Prescription drugs are the third leading cause of death," *The BMJ Opinion*, June 16, 2016, https://blogs.bmj.com/bmj/2016/06/16/peter-c-gotzsche-prescription-drugs-are-the-third-leading-cause-of-death/, accessed January 1, 2020.
7. "Acetaminophen/hydrocodone side-effects," www.drugs.com/sfx/acetaminophen-hydrocodone-side-effects.html, accessed January 3, 2020.
8. Abigail Davis and John Robson, "The dangers of NSAIDS: look both ways," *British Journal of General Practice*, April 2016; 66(645): 172–73, www.ncbi.nlm.nih.gov/pmc/articles/PMC4809680/, accessed January 2, 2020.
9. American Gastroentological Association, "Study shows long-term use of NSAIDs causes severe intestinal damage," *ScienceDaily*, January 16, 2005, www.sciencedaily.com/releases/2005/01/050111123706.htm, accessed January 2, 2020.
10. Felman, "What is pain?"
11. John M. Swegle et al., "Management of common opioid-induced adverse effects," *American Family Physician*, October 15, 2006; 74(8): 1347–54, www.aafp.org/afp/2006/1015/p1347.html, accessed January 12, 2020.
12. "Opioid (narcotic) pain medications," www.webmd.com/pain-management/guide/narcotic-pain-medications#1, accessed January 29, 2020.
13. Felman, "What is pain?"

14. Arthritis Foundation, "The Emotion-Pain Connection," www.arthritis.org /health-wellness/healthy-living/emotional-well-being/emotional-self-care/the -emotion-pain-connection, accessed January 12, 2020.

Chapter 2

1. "National statistics," www.cdc.gov/arthritis/data_statistics/national-statistics .html, accessed March 7, 2020.
2. "Back pain," www.mayoclinic.org/diseases-conditions/back-pain/symptoms -causes/syc-20369906, accessed March 7, 2020.
3. Ibid.
4. Ibid.
5. Ibid.
6. "Bursitis," www.mayoclinic.org/diseases-conditions/bursitis/symptoms-causes /syc-20353242, accessed March 7, 2020.
7. Ibid.
8. Ibid.
9. Ibid.
10. "Carpal tunnel syndrome," www.webmd.com/pain-management/carpal-tunnel /carpal-tunnel-syndrome#1, accessed March 2, 2020.
11. Ibid.
12. Angela Notarnicola et al., "Comparison of shock wave therapy and nutraceutical composed of *Echinacea angustifolia*, alpha lipoic acid, conjugated linoleic acid, and quercetin (perinerv) in patients with carpal tunnel syndrome," *International Journal of Immunopathology and Pharmacology*, June 2015; 28(2): 256–62, https://pubmed.ncbi.nlm.nih.gov/25953494/, accessed January 2, 2020.
13. "Peripheral neuropathy," www.mayoclinic.org/diseases-conditions/peripheral -neuropathy/symptoms-causes/syc-20352061, accessed February 1, 2020.
14. Ibid.
15. Ibid.
16. Ibid.
17. Kimberly Holland, "What you need to know about eye pain," www.healthline .com/symptom/eye-pain, accessed January 3, 2020.
18. American Chronic Pain Association, "Quick Facts on Fibromyalgia," www .theacpa.org/conditions-treatments/conditions-a-z/fibromyalgia/two-takes-on -fibro/quick-facts-on-fibromyalgia/, accessed January 14, 2020.
19. Stephanie Watson, "Signs and Symptoms of Fibromyalgia," www.healthline .com/health/fibromyalgia/signs-of-fibromyalgia, accessed January 4, 2020.
20. Miguel A. Pappolla et al., "Is insulin resistance the cause of fibromyalgia? A preliminary report," *PLOS One*, May 6, 2019, https://journals.plos.org/plosone /article?id=10.1371/journal.pone.0216079, accessed January 5, 2020.
21. William C. Shiel Jr, "Medical definition of insulin resistance," www.medicinenet .com/script/main/art.asp?articlekey=18822, accessed January 5, 2020.
22. "Apples," www.whfoods.com/genpage.php?tname=foodspice&dbid=15, accessed January 9, 2020.
23. Sonal Gupta Jain et al., "Effect of oral cinnamon intervention on metabolic profile and body composition of Asian Indians with metabolic syndrome: a randomized,

double-blind control trial," *Lipids in Health and Disease*, June 12, 2017; 16(1): 113, pubmed.ncbi.nlm.nih.gov/28606084/, accessed January 7, 2020.

24. Hassan Mozafarri-Khosravi et al., "The effect of ginger powder supplementation on insulin resistance and glycemic indices in patients with type 2 diabetes: a randomized, double-blind, placebo-controlled trial," *Complementary Therapies in Medicine*, February 2014; 22(1): 9–16, https://pubmed.ncbi.nlm.nih.gov/24559810/, accessed January 9, 2020.

25. Zhao-Qing Meng et al., "Study on the anti-gout activity of chlorogenic acid: study on hyperuricemia and gouty inflammation," *American Journal of Chinese Medicine*, 2014; 42(6):1471–83, https://pubmed.ncbi.nlm.nih.gov/25384446/, accessed June 2, 2020.

26. Robert Milne, Blake More, and Burton Goldberg, *An Alternative Medicine Definitive Guide to Headaches* (Tiburon, CA: Future Medicine, 1997), pp. 198–203.

27. Milne, More, and Goldberg, *Alternative Medicine Guide to Headaches*, pp. 198–203.

28. Anna Kokavec and Susan J. Crebbin, "Sugar alters the level of serum insulin and plasma glucose and the serum cortisol: DHEAS ratio in female migraine sufferers," *Appetite*, December 2010; 55(3): 582–88, https://pubmed.ncbi.nlm.nih.gov/20851729/?from_term=sugar+consumption+migraine&from_pos=3, accessed March 12, 2020.

29. Rajendrakumar M. Patel et al., "Popular sweetener sucralose as a migraine trigger," *Headache: The Journal of Head and Face Pain*, September 2006; 46(8): 1303–4, https://headachejournal.onlinelibrary.wiley.com/doi/full/10.1111/j.1526-4610.2006.00543_1.x, accessed January 17, 2020.

30. Anita Trauninger et al., "Oral magnesium load test in patients with migraine," *Headache: The Journal of Head and Face Pain*, February 2002; 42(2): 114–19, https://pubmed.ncbi.nlm.nih.gov/12005285/, accessed March 12, 2020.

31. Alexander Mauskop et al., "Serum ionized magnesium levels and serum ionized calcium/ionized magnesium ratios in women with menstrual migraine," *Headache: The Journal of Head and Face Pain*, April 2002; 42(4): 242–48, https://pubmed.ncbi.nlm.nih.gov/12010379/, accessed March 11, 2020.

32. Charly Gaul et al., "Improvement of migraine symptoms with a proprietary supplement containing riboflavin, magnesium, and Q10: a randomized, placebo-controlled, double-blind, multi-center trial," *Journal of Headache Pain*, 2015; 16: 516, https://pubmed.ncbi.nlm.nih.gov/25916335/, accessed March 9, 2020.

33. P. Sasannejad et al., "Lavender essential oil in the treatment of migraine headache: a placebo-controlled clinical trial," *European Neurology*, 2012; 67(5): 288–91, www.karger.com/Article/Abstract/335249, accessed November 27, 2020.

34. M. Niazi et al., "Efficacy of topical rose (*Rosa damascene* Mill.) oil for migraine headache: a randomized, double-blinded, placebo-controlled cross-over trial," *Complementary Therapies in Medicine*, October 2017; 34: 35–41, www.ncbi.nlm.nih.gov/pubmed/28917373, accessed November 27, 2020.

35. "UC researchers affirm diet can impact migraines," www.medicalnewstoday.com/mnt/releases/313850#1, accessed January 5, 2020.

36. Ann Pietrangelo, "Neck pain: possible causes and how to treat it," www.healthline.com/symptom/neck-pain, accessed April 22, 2020.

37. Ibid.

38. "Whiplash," Mayo Clinic, www.mayoclinic.org/diseases-conditions/whiplash/symptoms-causes/syc-20378921, accessed February 12, 2020.
39. "Plantar fasciitis," Mayo Clinic, www.mayoclinic.org/diseases-conditions/plantar-fasciitis/symptoms-causes/syc-20354846, accessed February 18, 2020.
40. Ibid.
41. Ibid.
42. Ibid.
43. Sabrina Hofmeister and Seth Bodden, "Premenstrual syndrome and premenstrual dysphoric disorder," *American Family Physician*, August 1, 2016; 94(3): 236–40, www.aafp.org/afp/2016/0801/p236.html, accessed January 27, 2020.
44. Patricia O. Chocano-Bedoyo et al., "Intake of selected minerals and risk of premenstrual syndrome," *American Journal of Epidemiology*, May 15, 2013; 177(10): 1118–27, https://academic.oup.com/aje/article/182/12/1000/2195531, accessed January 28, 2020.
45. "Sciatica," Mayo Clinic, www.mayoclinic.org/diseases-conditions/sciatica/symptoms-causes/syc-20377435, accessed January 28, 2020.
46. Ibid.
47. Ann Pietrangelo, "Why does my shoulder hurt?" www.healthline.com/health/chronic-pain/shoulder-pain, accessed January 30, 2020.
48. Ibid.
49. Ibid.
50. "Trigeminal neuralgia," www.mayoclinic.org/diseases-conditions/trigeminal-neuralgia/symptoms-causes/syc-20353344, accessed February 12, 2020.

Chapter 3

1. Stephanie Watson, "Autoimmune diseases: types, symptoms, causes, and more," www.healthline.com/health/autoimmune-disorders#bottom-line, accessed November 27, 2020. "Autoimmune disease list," www.aarda.org/diseaselist/, accessed November 27, 2020.
2. Ananya Mandal, "What are cytokines?" *NewsMedical*, May 17, 2014, www.news-medical.net/health/What-are-Cytokines.aspx, accessed November 27, 2020.
3. Alan C. Logan, *The Brain Diet* (Nashville, TN: Cumberland House, 2006), p. 114.
4. David M. Marquis, "How inflammation affects every aspect of your health," March 7, 2013, http://articles.mercola.com/sites/articles/archive/2013/03/07/inflammation-triggers-disease-symptoms.aspx, accessed November 27, 2020.
5. Ibid.
6. Ibid.
7. Eric M. Schott et al., "Targeting the gut microbiome to treat the osteoarthritis of obesity," *JCI Insight*, April 19, 2018, https://insight.jci.org/articles/view/95997, accessed March 1, 2020.
8. Jose U. Scher et al., "Expansion of intestinal *Prevotella copri* correlates with enhanced susceptibility to arthritis," *eLife*, November 5, 2013; 2: e01202, https://pubmed.ncbi.nlm.nih.gov/24192039/, accessed March 1, 2020.
9. Ibid.

10. Maria de Los Angeles Pineda et al., "A randomized, double-blind, placebo-controlled pilot study of probiotics in active rheumatoid arthritis," *Medical Science Monitor,* June 2011; 17(6): CR347–54, https://pubmed.ncbi.nlm.nih .gov/21629190/, accessed November 27, 2020.

11. Xiaofei Liu et al., "*Lactobacillus salivarius* isolated from patients with rheumatoid arthritis suppresses collagen-induced arthritis and increases Treg frequency in mice," *Journal of Interferon and Cytokine Research,* December 2016; 36(12): 706–12, https://pubmed.ncbi.nlm.nih.gov/27845855/, accessed February 29, 2020.

12. *The Probiotic Promise: Simple Steps to Heal Your Body from the Inside Out* (New York: DaCapo Lifelong Press, 2015).

13. Ashley Boynes Shuck, "Could balancing our gut bacteria be the key to unlocking RA?" www.healthline.com/health-news/could-balancing-gut-bacteria-be-key-to -unlocking-ra-012715#1, accessed March 3, 2020.

14. Hye-Ji Kang and Sin-Hyeog Im, "Probiotics as an immune modulator," *Journal of Nutritional Science and Vitaminology* (Tokyo), 2015; 61(suppl.): S103–5, www .ncbi.nlm.nih.gov/pubmed/26598815, accessed February 3, 2016.

15. Matteo M. Pusceddu and Melanie G. Gareau, "Visceral pain: gut microbiota, a new hope?" *Journal of Biomedical Science,* October 11, 2018; 25(1): 73, https:// pubmed.ncbi.nlm.nih.gov/30309367/, accessed March 12, 2020.

Chapter 4

1. Beverley Gray, *The Boreal Herbal: Wild Food and Medicine Plants of the North* (Whitehorse, YT: Aroma Borealis Press, 2011), p. 243.

2. Anna Fernandez, "Birch," www.herballegacy.com/Birch_History.html, accessed November 27, 2020.

3. Marie Miczak, *Nature's Weeds, Native Medicine: Native American Herbal Secrets* (Twin Lakes, WI: Lotus Press, 1999).

4. José Luis Ríos and Salvador Máñez, "New pharmacological opportunities for bet-ulinic acid," *Planta Medica,* January 2018; 84(1): 8–19, https://pubmed.ncbi.nlm .nih.gov/29202513/?from_term=birch+inflammation&from_pos=5, accessed November 27, 2020.

5. David Hoffmann, *Medical Herbalism: The Science and Practice of Herbal Medicine* (Rochester, VT: Healing Arts Press, 2003), p. 534.

6. David Young, Robert Robers, and Russell Willier, "Healing uses of sage and birch from a Cree healer and his medicinal bundle," June 1, 2015, www.north atlanticbooks.com/blog/healing-uses-of-sage-and-birch-from-a-cree-healer-and -his-medicine-bundle/, accessed November 27, 2020.

7. "Birch," www.webmd.com/vitamins/ai/ingredientmono-352/birch, accessed November 27, 2020.

8. Ibid.

9. James A. Duke, *The Green Pharmacy: The Ultimate Compendium of Natural Remedies from the World's Foremost Authority on Healing Herbs* (Emmaus, PA: Rodale Press), p. 547.

10. Hilary Parker, "What Causes Common Skin Warts?" www.webmd.com/skin -problems-and-treatments/features/viruses-cause-skin-warts#1, accessed November 27, 2020.

Chapter 5

1. Juliet Lapidos, "Readers respond to the editorial series on marijuana," *Taking Note, New York Times*, July 28, 2014, https://takingnote.blogs.nytimes.com/2014/07/28/readers-respond-to-the-editorial-series-on-marijuana/, accessed November 27, 2020.

2. Lindsay Stafford Mader, "The Quiet Giant: Israel's Discreet and Successful Medicinal Cannabis Program," http://cms.herbalgram.org/herbalgram/issue97/hg97-featcannabis.html?ts=1584645643&signature=038baf9d5534b35931c7f4b9ba0675e6&ts=1584645643&signature=0fa2ce3d3bc22646bc0be76ab2246972, accessed November 27, 2020.

3. UCLA Health, "Cannabis and its compounds," https://cannabis.semel.ucla.edu/compunds/, accessed December 1, 2020.

4. Health.com, "Medical marijuana for rheumatoid arthritis?" *Huffington Post*, June 8, 2011, www.huffpost.com/entry/can-medical-marijuana-help-arthritis_n_873189?guccounter=2, accessed November 27, 2020.

5. Christeene G. Haj et al., "HU-444, a novel, potent anti-inflammatory, non-psychotropic cannabinoid," *Journal of Pharmacology and Experimental Therapies*, October 2015; 335(1): 66–75, www.ncbi.nlm.nih.gov/pubmed/26272937, accessed November 27, 2020.

6. Health.com, "Medical marijuana for rheumatoid arthritis?"

7. Jody Corey-Bloom et al., "Smoked cannabis for plasticity in multiple sclerosis: a randomized, placebo-controlled trial," *CMAJ* (*Canadian Medical Association Journal*), July 10, 2012; 184(10): 1143–50, www.cmaj.ca/content/184/10/1143, accessed November 27, 2020.

8. Laszlo Mechtler et al., "Medical cannabis treatment in patients with trigeminal neuralgia," *Neurology*, April 16, 2019; 92(15 suppl.): p5.10-020, https://n.neurology.org/content/92/15_Supplement/P5.10-020, accessed November 27, 2020.

9. Alison Mack and Janet Joy, *Marijuana as Medicine? The Science Beyond the Controversy* (Washington, DC: National Academic Press, 2000), chap. 6, /www.ncbi.nlm.nih.gov/books/NBK224387/, accessed November 27, 2020.

10. Fred Cicetti, "How marijuana could help glaucoma," April 12, 2010, www.livescience.com/6232-marijuana-glaucoma.html, accessed November 27, 2020.

11. Caroline A. MacCallum and Ethan B. Russo, "Practical considerations in medical cannabis administration and dosing," *European Journal of Internal Medicine*, March 2018; 49: 12–19, www.ejinme.com/article/S0953-6205(18)30004-9/fulltext, accessed November 27, 2020.

12. Mark A. Ware et al., "Cannabis for the management of pain: assessment of safety study (COMPASS)," *Journal of Pain*, December 2015; 16(12): 1233–42, www.jpain.org/article/S1526-5900%2815%2900837-8/abstract, accessed November 27, 2020.

13. Centers for Disease Control and Prevention, "Outbreak of lung injury associated with the use of e-cigarette, or vaping, products," www.cdc.gov/tobacco/basic_information/e-cigarettes/severe-lung-disease.html, accessed November 27, 2020.

14. MacCallum and Russo, "Practical considerations in medical cannabis administration."

15. Cicetti, "How marijuana could help glaucoma."
16. UCLA Health, "Cannabis and its compounds," https://cannabis.semel.ucla.edu /compunds/, accessed December 1, 2020.
17. Lisa M. Eubanks et al., "A molecular link between the active component of marijuana and Alzheimer's disease pathology," *Molecular Pharmaceutics*, 2006; 3(6): 773–77, https://pubs.acs.org/doi/abs/10.1021/mp060066m?journalCode =mpohbp, accessed November 27, 2020.
18. Ed Susman, "Smoking pot eases tremors in Parkinson's," *MedPage Today*, January 18, 2013, www.medpagetoday.org/meetingcoverage/mds/39933?vpass=1, accessed November 27, 2020.
19. Robert J. DeLorenzo, "Marijuana and its receptor protein in brain control epilepsy," *VCU News*, March 31, 2020, www.news.vcu.edu/article/Marijuana_and _its_receptor_protein_in_brain_control_epilepsy, accessed November 27, 2020.
20. Sean D. McAllister et al., "Cannabidiol as a novel inhibitor of Id-1 gene expression in aggressive breast cancer cells," *Molecular Cancer Therapeutics*, November 2007; 6(11): 2921–27, www.ncbi.nlm.nih.gov/pubmed/18025276, accessed November 27, 2020.

Chapter 6

1. James A. Duke, PhD, *The Green Pharmacy: The Ultimate Compendium of Natural Remedies from the World's Foremost Authority on Healing Herbs* (Emmaus, PA: Rodale Press Inc., 1997), pg. 272.
2. Michael C. Powanda et al., "Celery seed and related extracts with antiarthritic, antiulcer, and antimicrobial activities," *Progress in Drug Research*, 2015; 70: 133– 53, www.ncbi.nlm.nih.gov/pubmed/26462366, accessed November 27, 2020.
3. Shaopeng Li et al., "Anti-gouty arthritis and anti-hyperuricemia properties of celery seed extracts in rodent models," *Molecular Medicine Reports*, November 2019; 20(5): 4623–33, www.ncbi.nlm.nih.gov/pubmed/31702020, accessed November 27, 2020.

Chapter 7

1. Sheena Derry, "Topical capsaicin (high concentration) for chronic neuropathic pain in adults," *Cochrane Database of Systematic Reviews*, February 28, 2013; (2): CD007393, www.ncbi.nlm.nih.gov/pubmed/23450576, accessed November 27, 2020.
2. David Hoffmann, *Medical Herbalism: The Science and Practice of Herbal Medicine* (Rochester, VT: Healing Arts Press, 2003), p. 536.
3. Ibid.
4. Hanna Oltean et al., "Herbal medicine for low back pain," *Cochrane Database of Systematic Reviews*, December 23, 2014; (12): CD004504, www.ncbi.nlm.nih .gov/pubmed/25536022, accessed November 27, 2020.
5. L. Limlomwongse et al., "Effect of capsaicin on gastric acid secretion and mucosal blood flow in the rat," *Journal of Nutrition*, 1979; 109: 773–77. O. Ketusinh et al., "Influence of capsaicin solution on gastric acidities," *American Journal of Proctology* 1966; 17: 511–15, https://europepmc.org/article/med/5980698.

Chapter 8

1. "History of cloves," www.indepthinfo.com/cloves/story.shtml, accessed November 27, 2020.
2. Tash Penman, "The complete list of ORAC ratings for essential oils," www.theresaneoforthat.com/the-complete-list-of-orac-ratings-for-essential-oils/, accessed November 27, 2020.
3. Kurt Schnaubelt, *Advanced Aromatherapy: The Science of Essential Oil Therapy* (Rochester, VT: Healing Arts Press, 1995), p. 65.
4. Jose U. Scher et al., "Expansion of intestinal *Prevotella copri* correlates with enhanced susceptibility to arthritis," *eLife*, November 5, 2013; 2: e01202, https://pubmed.ncbi.nlm.nih.gov/24192039/, accessed March 1, 2020.
5. Athbi Alqareer et al., "The effect of clove and benzocaine versus placebo as topical anesthetics," *Journal of Dentistry*, November 2006; 34(10): 747–50, www.sciencedirect.com/science/article/pii/S0300571206000248, accessed November 27, 2020.
6. Zheng Tu et al., "*Syzygium aromaticum* L. (clove) extract regulates energy metabolism in myocytes," *Journal of Medicinal Food*, September 2014; 17(9): 1003–10, www.ncbi.nlm.nih.gov/pubmed/24999964, accessed November 27, 2020.

Chapter 9

1. Amelia Meyer, "The Amazon rainforest," www.brazil.org.za/amazon-rainforest.html, accessed November 27, 2020.
2. Leslie Taylor, "Copaiba," www.rain-tree.com/copaiba.htm, accessed November 27, 2020.
3. R. La Roche, "Dr. La Roche on copaiba in bronchitis," www.ncbi.nlm.nih.gov/pmc/articles/PMC5674635/pdf/londmedphysj74712-0011.pdf, accessed November 27, 2020.
4. "Dr. Hill discusses copaiba and cannabinoid benefits," www.youtube.com/watch?v=axmJurEhptY&list=PLp3VbOdUkkm3j-E47KpJ_t9vnwqqcvubB&index=9&fbclid=IwAR3zYaAMMUuxKFbm29lbht3U8LUwoG7kipXiz8OtXZX1i0op4bSPK0a0Qnc, accessed November 27, 2020.
5. Tyler Strause, "7 things you probably didn't know about the endocannabinoid system," https://medium.com/randy-s-club/7-things-you-probably-didnt-know-about-the-endocannabinoid-system-35e264c802bc, accessed November 27, 2020.
6. "Dr. Hill discusses copaiba and cannabinoid benefits." Strause, "7 things about the endocannabinoid system."
7. Dustin Sulak, "Introduction to the Endocannabinoid System," https://norml.org/library/item/introduction-to-the-endocannabinoid-system, accessed November 27, 2020.
8. "Dr. Hill discusses copaiba and cannabinoid benefits."
9. "Dr. Hill discusses copaiba and cannabinoid benefits."
10. Ana P. Ames-Sibin et al., "β-caryophyllene, the major constituent of copaiba oil, reduces systemic inflammation and oxidative stress in arthritic rats," *Journal of Cellular Biochemistry*, December 2018; 119(12): 10262–77, www.ncbi.nlm.nih.gov/pubmed/30132972, accessed November 27, 2020.

11. Tyler Bahr et al., "Effects of a massage-like oil application procedure using copaiba and Deep Blue oils in individuals with hand arthritis," *Complementary Therapy in Clinical Practice*, November 2018; 33: 170–76, www.ncbi.nlm.nih .gov/pubmed/30396617, accessed November 27, 2020.
12. Taylor, "Copaiba."
13. Taylor, "Copaiba."
14. Guifang Wang et al., "β-caryophyllene (BCP) ameliorates MPP+ induced cyto- toxicity," *Biomedicine & Pharmacotherapy*, July 2018; 103: 1086–91, www.ncbi .nlm.nih.gov/pubmed/?term=B-Caryophyllene+(BCP)+ameliorates+MPP %2B+induced+cytotoxicity, accessed November 27, 2020.
15. Taylor, "Copaiba."
16. Pál Pacher et al., "The endocannabinoid system as an emerging target of pharma- cotherapy," *Pharmacological Reviews*, September 2006; 58(3): 389–462, www .ncbi.nlm.nih.gov/pmc/articles/PMC2241751/, accessed November 27, 2020.

Chapter 10

1. Mark Blumenthal et al., *The Complete German Commission E Monographs* (Aus- tin, TX: American Botanical Council, 1998).
2. Tankred Wegener and Niels-Peter Lüpke, "Treatment of patients with arthrosis of hip or knee with an aqueous extract of devil's claw (*Harpagophytum procum- bens* DC.)," *Phytotherapy Research* 2003; 17: 1165–72, www.ncbi.nlm.nih.gov /pubmed/14669250, accessed November 27, 2020. P. Chantre et al., "Efficacy and tolerance of *Harpagophytum procumbens* versus diacerhein in treatment of osteoarthritis," *Phytomedicine* 2000; 7: 177–83, https://pubmed.ncbi.nlm.nih .gov/11185727, accessed Noember 27, 2020.
3. Rachel Brakke, "What is crepitus?" www.arthritis-health.com/types/general /what-crepitus, accessed November 27, 2020.
4. S. Chrubasik et al., "Comparison of outcome measures during treatment with the proprietary *Harpagophytum* extract Doloteffin in patients with pain in the lower back, knee, or hip," *Phytomedicine*, 2002; 9: 181–94, https://pubmed.ncbi.nlm .nih.gov/12046857/, accessed November 27, 2020.
5. B. L. Fiebich et al., "Inhibition of TNF-alpha synthesis in LPS-stimulated pri- mary human monocytes by *Harpagophytum* extract SteiHap 69," *Phytomedi- cine*, 2001; 8(1): 28–30, https://pubmed.ncbi.nlm.nih.gov/11292236/, accessed November 27, 2020.
6. Nontobeko Mncwangi et al., "Devil's claw—a review of the ethnobotany, phyto- chemistry, and biological activity of *Harpagophytum procumbens*," *Journal of Ethnopharmacology*, October 11, 2012; 143(3): 755–71, www.ncbi.nlm.nih.gov /pubmed/22940241, accessed November 27, 2020.
7. M. C. Lanhers et al., "Anti-inflammatory and analgesic effects of an aqueous extract of *Harpagophytum procumbens*," *Planta Medica*, April 1992; 58(2): 117– 23, pubmed.ncbi.nlm.nih.gov/1529021/, accessed November 27, 2020.
8. "Devil's claw," www.webmd.com/vitamins-supplements/ingredientmono-984 -DEVIL'S%20CLAW.aspx?activeIngredientId=984&activeIngredientName =DEVIL%27S%20CLAW, accessed November 27, 2020.
9. Marcello Locatelli et al., "Optimization of aqueous extraction and biological activity of *Harpagophytum procumbens* root on ex vivo rat colon inflammatory

model," *Phytotherapy Research*, June 2017; 31(6): 937–44, https://pubmed.ncbi
.nlm.nih.gov/28447368/?from_term=harpagophytum+procumbens&from_pos
=2, accessed November 27, 2020.

Chapter 11

1. David Hoffmann, *Medical Herbalism: The Science and Practice of Herbal Medicine* (Rochester, VT: Healing Arts Press, 2003), p. 550.
2. Roman Paduch et al., "Assessment of eyebright (*Euphrasia officinalis* L.) extract activity in relation to human corneal cells using in vitro tests," *Balkan Medical Journal*, March 2014; 31(1): 29–36, https://pubmed.ncbi.nlm.nih.gov /25207164/?from_term=euphrasia+officinalis&from_pos=4, accessed November 27, 2020.
3. Elisabetta Bigagli et al., "Pharmacological activities of an eye drop containing *Matricaria chamomilla* and *Euphrasia officinalis* extracts in UVB-induced oxidative stress and inflammation of human corneal cells," *Journal of Photochemistry and Photobiology B: Biology*, August 2017; 173: 618–25, https://pubmed .ncbi.nlm.nih.gov/28704790/?from_term=euphrasia+officinalis&from_pos=3, accessed November 27, 2020.
4. M. Stoss et al., "Prospective cohort trial of *Euphrasia* single-dose eye drops in conjunctivitis," *Journal of Alternative and Complementary Medicine*, December 2000; 6(6): 499–508, https://pubmed.ncbi.nlm.nih.gov/11152054/?from_single _result=euphrasia+Witwatersrand&expanded_search_query=euphrasia +Witwatersrand, accessed November 27, 2020.

Chapter 12

1. *The Essential Life: The World's Most Trusted Essential Oil Reference Guide*, 6th ed. (Pleasant Grove, UT: Total Wellness, 2019), p. 109.
2. S. N. Ostad et al., "The effect of fennel essential oil on uterine contraction as a model for dysmenorrhea, pharmacology and toxicology study," *Journal of Ethnopharmacology*, August 2001; 76(3): 299–304, www.ncbi.nlm.nih.gov /pubmed/11448553, accessed November 27, 2020.
3. Masoomeh Nasehi et al., "Comparison of the effectiveness of combination of fennel extract/vitamin E with ibuprofen on the pain intensity in students with primary dysmenorrhea," *Iranian Journal of Nursing and Midwifery Research*, September–October 2013; 18(5): 355–59, www.ncbi.nlm.nih.gov/pmc/articles /PMC3877456/, accessed November 27, 2020.

Chapter 13

1. Barbara Wider et al., "Feverfew for preventing migraine," *Cochrane Database of Systematic Reviews*, April 20, 2015; 4(4): CD002286, www.ncbi.nlm.nih.gov /pubmed/25892430, accessed March 14, 2020.
2. Lorenzo Di Cesare Mannelli et al., "Widespread pain reliever profile of a flower extract of *Tanacetum parthenium*," *Phytomedicine*, July 15, 2015; 22(7–8): 752–58, www.ncbi.nlm.nih.gov/pubmed/26141762, accessed March 12, 2020.

3. David Hoffmann, *Medical Herbalism: The Science and Practice of Herbal Medicine* (Rochester, VT: Healing Arts Press, 2003), p. 587.
4. Ibid.

Chapter 14

1. Ahmed Al-Harrasi et al., "Analgesic effects of crude extracts and fractions of Omani frankincense obtained from traditional medicinal plant *Boswellia sacra* on animal models," *Asian Pacific Journal of Tropical Medicine*, September 2014; 7S1: S485–90, www.ncbi.nlm.nih.gov/pubmed/25312172, accessed March 1, 2020.
2. Muhammed Majeed et al., "A pilot, randomized, double-blind, placebo-controlled trial to assess the safety and efficacy of a novel *Boswellia serrata* extract in the management of osteoarthritis of the knee," *Phytotherapy Research*, May 2019; 33(5): 1457–68, www.ncbi.nlm.nih.gov/pmc/articles/PMC6681146/, accessed March 12, 2020.
3. G. Bolognesi et al., "Movardol® (N-acetylglucosamine, *Boswellia serrata*, ginger) supplementation in the management of knee osteoarthritis: preliminary results from a 6-month registry study," *European Review for Medical and Pharmacological Sciences*, December 2016; 20(24): 5198–204, https://pubmed.ncbi.nlm.nih.gov/28051248/, accessed March 10, 2020.
4. G. Merolla et al., "Co-analgesic therapy for arthroscopic supraspinatus tendon repair pain using a dietary supplement containing *Boswellia serrata* and *Curcuma longa*: a prospective, randomized, placebo-controlled study," *Musculoskeletal Surgery*, September 2015; 99(suppl. 1): S43–52, https://pubmed.ncbi.nlm.nih.gov/25957549/, accessed March 10, 2020.
5. G. Bolognesi et al., "Movardol® (N-acetylglucosamine, *Boswellia serrata*, ginger) supplementation in the management of knee osteoarthritis."
6. "Definition and facts for irritable bowel syndrome," www.niddk.nih.gov/health-information/digestive-diseases/irritable-bowel-syndrome/definition-facts, accessed March 12, 2020.
7. Arieh Moussaieff et al., "Incensole acetate reduces depressive-like behavior and modulates hippocampal BDNF and CRF expression of submissive animals," *Journal of Psychopharmacology*, December 2012; 26(12): 1584–93, www.ncbi.nlm.nih.gov/pubmed/23015543, accessed March 6, 2020.
8. *Modern Essentials: A Contemporary Guide to the Therapeutic Use of Essential Oils* (Pleasant Grove, UT: AromaTools, 2016), p. 63.

Chapter 15

1. Søren Ribel-Madsen et al., "A synoviocyte model for osteoarthritis and rheumatoid arthritis: response to ibuprofen, betamethasone, and ginger extract—a cross-sectional in vitro study," *Arthritis*, 2012; 2012: 505842, www.ncbi.nlm.nih.gov/pubmed/23365744, accessed March 1, 2020.
2. R. D. Altman and K. C. Marcussen, "Effect of a ginger extract on knee pain in patients with osteoarthritis," *Arthritis and Rheumatism*, November 2001; 44(11): 2531–38, www.ncbi.nlm.nih.gov/pubmed/11710709, accessed November 27, 2020.

3. Vladimir N. Drozdov et al., "Influence of a specific ginger combination on gastropathy conditions in patients with osteoarthritis of the knee or hip," *Journal of Alternative and Complementary Medicine*, June 2012; 18(6): 583–88, www .ncbi.nlm.nih.gov/pubmed/22784345, accessed November 27, 2020.
4. Ribel-Madsen et al., "A synoviocyte model for osteoarthritis and rheumatoid arthritis."
5. K. C. Srivastava and T. Mustafa, "Ginger (*Zingiber officinalis*) in rheumatism and musculoskeletal disorders," *Medical Hypotheses*, December 1992; 39(4): 342–48, www.ncbi.nlm.nih.gov/pubmed/1494322, accessed November 27, 2020.
6. Ibid.
7. Ibid.

Chapter 16

1. "Lavender," www.cs.mcgill.ca/~rwest/wikispeedia/wpcd/wp/l/Lavender.htm, accessed March 2, 2020.
2. Ibid.
3. Tamaki Matsumoto et al., "Does lavender aromatherapy alleviate premenstrual emotional symptoms? A randomized crossover trial," *BioPsychoSocial Medicine*, May 31, 2013; 7: 12, www.ncbi.nlm.nih.gov/pubmed/23724853, accessed November 27, 2020.
4. Monsoreh Yazdkhasti and Arezoo Pirak, "The effect of aromatherapy with lavender essence on severity of labor pain and duration of labor in primiparous women," *Complementary Therapies in Clinical Practice*, November 2016; 25: 81–86, https://pubmed.ncbi.nlm.nih.gov/27863615/?from_term=lavandula +angustifolia+pain&from_pos=4, accessed February 12, 2020.
5. Maria Domenica Sanna et al., "Lavender (*Lavandula angustifolia* Mill.) essential oil alleviates neuropathic pain in mice with spared nerve injury," *Frontiers in Pharmacology*, May 9, 2019; 10: 472, https://pubmed.ncbi.nlm.nih.gov/31143116 /?from_term=lavandula+angustifolia+pain&from_pos=1, accessed February 12, 2020.
6. Nathalia Nahas Donatello et al., "*Lavandula angustifolia* essential oil inhalation reduces mechanical hyperalgesia in a model of inflammatory and neuropathic pain: the involvement of opioid and cannabinoid receptors," *Journal of Neuro-immunology*, March 15, 2020; 340: 577145, https://linkinghub.elsevier.com /retrieve/pii/S0165572819304436, accessed March 15, 2020.
7. Ahmad Nasiri et al., "Effect of aromatherapy massage with lavender essential oil on pain in patients with osteoarthritis of the knee: a randomized controlled clinical trial," *Complementary Therapies in Clinical Practice*, November 2016; 25: 75–80, www.sciencedirect.com/science/article/abs/pii/S1744388116300597?via %3Dihub, accessed March 1, 2020.
8. Katayon Vakilian et al., "Healing advantages of lavender essential oil during episiotomy recovery: a clinical trial," *Complementary Therapies in Clinical Practice*, February 2011; 17(1): 50–53, www.sciencedirect.com/science/article/abs/pii /S1744388110000381, accessed November 27, 2020.
9. H. M. A. Cavanagh and J. M. Wilkinson, "Biological activities of lavender essential oil," *Phytotherapy Research*, June 2002; 16(4): 301–8, https://pubmed.ncbi .nlm.nih.gov/12112282/, accessed November 27, 2020.

10. Masoud Nikfarjam et al., "The effects of *Lavandula angustifolia* Mill infusion on depression in patients using citalopram: a comparison study," *Iranian Red Crescent Medical Journal*, August 2013; 15(8): 734–39, www.ncbi.nlm.nih.gov /pubmed/24578844, accessed November 27, 2020.

Chapter 17

1. Joshua J. Kang et al., "Comparative anti-inflammatory effects of anti-arthritic herbal medicines and ibuprofen," *Natural Product Communications*, September 2014; 9(9): 1351–56, www.ncbi.nlm.nih.gov/pubmed/25918809, accessed January 2020.
2. Ke-feng Zhai et al., "Liquiritin from *Glycyrrhiza uralensis* attenuating rheumatoid arthritis via reducing inflammation, suppressing angiogenesis, and inhibiting MAPK signaling pathway," *Journal of Agricultural and Food Chemistry*, March 13, 2019; 67(10): 2586–64, https://pubs.acs.org/doi/10.1021/acs.jafc.9b00185, accessed January 3, 2020.
3. Rui Yang et al., "The anti-inflammatory activity of licorice, a widely used Chinese herb," *Pharmaceutical Biology*, 2017; 55(1): 5–18, www.tandfonline.com /doi/full/10.1080/13880209.2016.1225775, accessed January 2, 2020.
4. Daniel B. Mowrey, PhD, *The Scientific Validation of Herbal Medicine: How to Remedy and Prevent Disease with Herbs, Vitamins, Minerals, and Other Nutrients*, (Los Angeles: Keats Publishing, 1986).
5. John F. Rebhun et al., "Identification of glabridin as a bioactive compound in licorice (*Glycyrrhiza glabra* L.) extract that activates human peroxisome proliferator-activated receptor gamma (PPARγ)," *Fitoterapia*, October 2015; 106: 55–61, www.ncbi.nlm.nih.gov/pubmed/26297329, accessed January 1, 2020.
6. Fei Jiang et al., "Glabridin inhibits cancer stem cell-like properties of human breast cancer cells: an epigenetic regulation of miR-148a/SMAd2 signaling," *Molecular Carcinogenesis*, May 2016; 55(5): 929–40, www.ncbi.nlm.nih.gov /pubmed/25980823, accessed January 2, 2020.

Chapter 18

1. *The Essential Life: The World's Most Trusted Essential Oil Reference Guide*, 6th ed. (Pleasant Grove, UT: Total Wellness, 2019), p. 113.
2. Gabriel Mojay, *Aromatherapy for Healing the Spirit: Restoring Emotional and Mental Balance with Essential Oils* (Rochester, VT: Healing Arts Press, 1997), p. 94.
3. Ibid.
4. Hanane Makrane et al., "Myorelaxant activity of essential oil from *Origanum majorana* L. on rat and rabbit," *Journal of Ethnopharmacology*, January 10, 2019; 228: 40–49, https://pubmed.ncbi.nlm.nih.gov/30205180/?from_term=origanum +majorana&from_pos=3, accessed January 7, 2020.
5. Ming-Chiu Ou et al., "Pain relief assessment by aromatic essential oil massage on outpatients with primary dysmenorrhea: a randomized, double-blind, clinical trial," *Journal of Obstetrics and Gynaecology Research*, May 2012; 38(5): 817–22, https://doi.org/10.1111/j.1447-0756.2011.01802.x, accessed January 28, 2020.

6. Ming-Chiu Ou et al., "The effectiveness of essential oils for patients with neck pain: a randomized controlled study," *Journal of Alternative and Complementary Medicine*, October 9, 2014; 20(10): 771–79, www.liebertpub.com/doi/10.1089/acm.2013.0453, accessed January 13, 2020.
7. Fatemeh Bina and Roja Rahimi, "Sweet marjoram: a review of ethnopharmacology, phytochemistry, and biological activities," *Journal of Evidence-Based Complementary and Alternative Medicine*, January 2017; 22(1): 175–85, www.ncbi.nlm.nih.gov/pmc/articles/PMC5871212/#bibr8-2156587216650793, accessed January 11, 2020.
8. *The Essential Life*, p. 131.
9. John F. Carroll et al., "Repellency of the *Origanum onites* L. essential oil and constituents to the lone star tick and yellow fever mosquito," *Natural Product Research*, September 2017; 31(18): 2192–97, www.ncbi.nlm.nih.gov/pubmed/28278656, accessed January 12, 2020.

Chapter 19

1. Lumir O. Hanus et al., "Myrrh—*Commiphora* chemistry," *Biomed Papers*, 2005; 149(1): 3–28, http://biomed.papers.upol.cz/pdfs/bio/2005/01/01.pdf, accessed February 2020.
2. Antonio Germano et al., "A pilot study on bioactive constituents and analgesic effects of MyrLiq®, a *Commiphora myrrha* extract with a high furanodiene content," *BioMed Research International*, 2017; 2017: 3804356, https://pubmed.ncbi.nlm.nih.gov/28626756/, accessed March 12, 2020.
3. Leonardo Scarzella, "Effects of a novel MyrLiq®, *Ginkgo biloba*, Q10, and vitamin B2 (riboflavin) based nutraceutical in patients suffering from migraine headache without aura or sporadic episodes of tension-type headache: a six-month pilot study," *Gazetta Medica Italiana Archivio per le Scienze Mediche*, April 2017; 176(4): 149–53, www.minervamedica.it/en/journals/gazzetta-medica-italiana/article.php?cod=R22Y2017N04A0149, accessed March 6, 2020.
4. Marsha McCulloch, "11 surprising uses and benefits of myrrh oil," www.healthline.com/nutrition/myrrh-oil, accessed March 1, 2020.
5. Shulan Su et al., "Anti-inflammatory and analgesic activity of different extracts of *Commiphora Myrrha*," *Journal of Ethnopharmacology*, March 24, 2011; 134(2): 251–58, https://pubmed.ncbi.nlm.nih.gov/21167270/, accessed March 1, 2020.
6. Dai Mizuno et al., "An in vitro system comprising immortalized hypothalamic neuronal cells (GT1-7 cells) for evaluation of the neuroendocrine effects of essential oils," *Evidence-Based Complementary and Alternative Medicine*, 2015; 2015: 343942, www.ncbi.nlm.nih.gov/pubmed/26576190, accessed February 12, 2020.
7. Uppuluri Venkata Mallavadhani et al., "Synthesis and anticancer activity of novel fused pyrimidine hybrids of myrrhanone C, a bicyclic triterpene of *Commiphora mukul* gum resin," *Molecular Diversity*, November 2015; 19(4): 745–57, www.ncbi.nlm.nih.gov/pubmed/26232027, accessed November 27, 2020.
8. Ajaz A. Bhat, et al., "Potential therapeutic targets of guggulsterone in cancer," *Nutrition and Metabolism* (London), February 28, 2017; 14:23, https://pubmed.ncbi.nlm.nih.gov/28261317/, accessed December 1, 2020.

Chapter 20

1. "Oregano," www.indepthinfo.com/oregano/history.shtml, accessed November 27, 2020.
2. Adriana G. Guimarães et al., "Carvacrol attenuates mechanical hypernociception and inflammatory response," *Naunyn-Schmiedeberg's Archives of Pharmacology*, 2012; 385: 253–63, https://link.springer.com/article/10.1007/s00210-011-0715-x, accessed January 7, 2020.
3. Juliane C. Silva et al., "Enhancement of orofacial antinociceptive effect of carvacrol, a monoterpene present in oregano and thyme oils, by β-cyclodextrin inclusion complex in mice," *Biomedicine & Pharmacotherapy*, December 2016; 84: 454–61, www.sciencedirect.com/science/article/abs/pii/S0753332216311076?via%3Dihub, accessed January 8, 2020.
4. Gloria Magi et al., "Antimicrobial activity of essential oils and carvacrol, and synergy of carvacrol and erythromycin, against clinical, erythromycin-resistant, Group A streptococci," *Frontiers in Microbiology*, March 3, 2015; 6: 165, www.ncbi.nlm.nih.gov/pubmed/25784902, accessed November 27, 2020.
5. Karine Rech Begnini et al., "Composition and antiproliferative effect of essential oil of *Origanum vulgare* against tumor cell lines," *Journal of Medicinal Food*, October 2014; 17(10): 1129–33, www.ncbi.nlm.nih.gov/pubmed/25230257, accessed November 27, 2020.
6. Mariangela Marrelli et al., "Inhibitory effects of wild dietary plants on lipid peroxidation and on the proliferation of human cancer cells," *Food and Chemical Toxicology*, December 2015; 86: 16–24, www.ncbi.nlm.nih.gov/pubmed/26408343, accessed November 27, 2020.

Chapter 21

1. "Peppermint," www.whfoods.com/genpage.php?tname=foodspice&dbid=102, accessed November 27, 2020.
2. Ming-Chiu Ou et al., "The effectiveness of essential oils for patients with neck pain: a randomized controlled study," *Journal of Alternative and Complementary Medicine*, October 2014; 20(10): 771–79, www.liebertpub.com/doi/10.1089/acm.2013.0453, accessed January 13, 2020.
3. Andrea St. Cyr et al., "Efficacy and tolerability of STOPain for a migraine attack," *Frontiers in Neurology*, 2015; 6: 11, www.ncbi.nlm.nih.gov/pmc/articles/PMC4316718/, accessed January 18, 2020.
4. H. G. Grigoleit and P. Grigoleit, "Peppermint oil in irritable bowel syndrome," *Phytomedicine*, August 2005; 12(8): 601–6, https://pubmed.ncbi.nlm.nih.gov/30423929/, January 14, 2020.
5. Mohaddese Mahboubi, "Caraway as important medicinal plants in management of diseases," *Natural Products and Bioprospecting*, February 2019; 9(1): 1–11, www.ncbi.nlm.nih.gov/pmc/articles/PMC6328425/, accessed January 15, 2020.
6. Jill Seladi-Schulman, "About peppermint oil uses and benefits," www.healthline.com/health/benefits-of-peppermint-oil#gi-pain, accessed February 1, 2020.
7. A. Schumacher et al., "Virucidal effect of peppermint oil on the enveloped viruses herpes simplex virus type 1 and type 2 in vitro," *Phytomedicine*, 2003; 10(6–7): 504–10, www.ncbi.nlm.nih.gov/pubmed/13678235, accessed November 27, 2020.

Chapter 22

1. James A. Duke, *The Green Pharmacy: The Ultimate Compendium of Natural Remedies from the World's Foremost Authority on Healing Herbs* (Emmaus, PA: Rodale Press).
2. Beth Dunn, "A Brief History of Thyme," www.history.com/news/a-brief-history -of-thyme, accessed February 13, 2020.
3. Adriana G. Guimarães et al., "Carvacrol attenuates mechanical hypernociception and inflammatory response," *Naunyn-Schmiedeberg's Archives of Pharmacology*, 2012; 385: 253–63, https://link.springer.com/article/10.1007/s00210-011-0715-x, accessed January 7, 2020.
4. Juliane C. Silva et al., "Enhancement of orofacial antinociceptive effect of carvacrol, a monoterpene present in oregano and thyme oils, by β-cyclodextrin inclusion complex in mice," *Biomedicine & Pharmacotherapy*, December 2016; 84: 454–61, www.sciencedirect.com/science/article/abs/pii/S0753332216311076?via %3Dihub, accessed January 8, 2020.
5. "Aspergillosis," www.cdc.gov/fungal/diseases/aspergillosis/index.html?s_cid=cs _748, accessed January 26, 2020.
6. Mohd S. A. Khan et al., "*Carum coptum* and *Thymus vulgaris* oils inhibit virulence in *Trichophyton rubrum* and *Aspergillus* spp," *Brazilian Journal of Microbiology*, August 29, 2014; 45(2): 523–31, www.ncbi.nlm.nih.gov/pubmed/25242937, accessed January 25, 2020.
7. Mohd S. A. Khan et al., "Sub-MICs of *Carum copticum* and *Thymus vulgaris* influence virulence factors and biofilm formation in *Candida* spp," *BMC Complementary and Alternative Medicine*, September 15, 2014; 14: 337, www.ncbi.nlm .nih.gov/pubmed/25220750, accessed January 12, 2020.

Chapter 23

1. Constanze Buhrmann et al., "Curcumin moderates nuclear factor kappaB (NF-kappaB)-mediated inflammation in human tenocytes in vitro: role of the phosphatidylinositol 3-kinase/Akt pathway," *Journal of Biological Chemistry*, August 12, 2011; 286(32): 28556–66, www.ncbi.nlm.nih.gov/pubmed/21669872, accessed November 27, 2020.
2. Yasunari Takada et al., "Nonsteroidal anti-inflammatory agents differ in their ability to suppress NF-kappaB activation, inhibition of expression of cyclooxygenase-2 and cyclin D1, and abrogation of tumor cell proliferation," *Oncogene*, December 9, 2004; 23(57): 9247–58, www.ncbi.nlm.nih.gov/pubmed/15489888, accessed November 27, 2020.
3. Francesco Di Pierro et al., "Comparative evaluation of the pain-relieving properties of a lecithinized formulation of curcumin (Meriva(®)), nimesulide, and acetaminophen," *Journal of Pain Research*, 2013, https://pubmed.ncbi.nlm.nih .gov/23526055/, accessed December 1, 2020.
4. Franchek Drobnik et al., "Reduction of delayed onset muscle soreness by a novel curcumin delivery system (Meriva®): a randomised, placebo-controlled trial," *Journal of the International Society of Sports Nutrition*, 2014; 11: 31, www.jissn .com/content/11/1/31, accessed November 27, 2020.

5. Mina Cheraghi Nirumand et al., "Dietary plants for the prevention and management of kidney stones: preclinical and clinical evidence and molecular mechanisms," *International Journal of Molecular Sciences*, March 7, 2018; 19(3): 765, www.ncbi.nlm.nih.gov/pubmed/29518971, accessed November 27, 2020.
6. Vilai Kuptniratsaikul et al., "Efficacy and safety of *Curcuma domestica* extracts compared with ibuprofen in patients with knee osteoarthritis: a multicenter study," *Clinical Interventions in Aging*, March 20, 2014; 9: 451–58, www.ncbi.nlm.nih.gov/pubmed/24672232, accessed March 1, 2020.
7. Namyata Pathak-Gandhi and Ashok D. B. Vaidya, "Management of Parkinson's Disease in Ayurveda: medicinal plants and adjuvant measures," *Journal of Ethnopharmacology*, February 2, 2017; 197: 46–51, www.sciencedirect.com/science/article/pii/S0378874116305463?via%3Dihub, accessed November 27, 2020.
8. Joerg Hucklenbroich et al., "Aromatic-turmerone induces neural stem cell proliferation in vitro and in vivo," *Stem Cell Research & Therapy*, September 26, 2014; 5(4): 100, www.ncbi.nlm.nih.gov/pubmed/25928248, accessed March 3, 2020.
9. Dong-Wei Zhang et al., "Curcumin and diabetes: a systematic review," *Evidence-Based Complementary and Alternative Medicine*, 2013; 2013: 636053, https://pubmed.ncbi.nlm.nih.gov/24348712/, accessed March 1, 2020.
10. Katherine H. M. Cox et al., "Investigation of the effects of a solid lipid curcumin on cognition and mood in a healthy older population," *Journal of Psychopharmacology*, May 2015; 29(5): 642–51, www.ncbi.nlm.nih.gov/pubmed/25277322, accessed February 1, 2020.
11. "Curry ingredient may stop Alzheimer's," www.medicalnewstoday.com/releases/13116, accessed January 5, 2020.
12. Nozomi Hishikawa et al., "Effects of turmeric on Alzheimer's disease with behavioral and psychological symptoms of dementia," *AYU*, October 2012; 33(4): 499–504, www.ncbi.nlm.nih.gov/pubmed/23723666, accessed January 29, 2020.

Chapter 24

1. David Hoffmann, *Medical Herbalism: The Science and Practice of Herbal Medicine* (Rochester, VT: Healing Arts Press, 2003), p. 579.
2. Mohd Shara and Sidney J. Stohs, "Efficacy and safety of white willow bark (*Salix alba*) extracts," *Phytotherapy Research*, August 2015; 29(8): 1112–16, https://pubmed.ncbi.nlm.nih.gov/25997859/, accessed March 12, 2020.
3. Z. Raisi Dehkoordi et al., "A double-blind, controlled, cross-over study to investigate the efficacy of salix extract on primary dysmenorrhea," *Complementary Therapies in Medicine*, June 2019; 44: 102–9, https://pubmed.ncbi.nlm.nih.gov/31126541/, accessed March 10, 2020.
4. Hanna Oltean et al., "Herbal medicine for low-back pain," *Cochrane Database of Systematic Reviews*, December 23, 2014; 2014(12): CD004504, https://pubmed.ncbi.nlm.nih.gov/25536022/, accessed February 28, 2020.
5. Shara and Stohs, "Efficacy and safety of white willow bark extracts."
6. Hoffmann, *Medical Herbalism*, p. 579.
7. Oltean et al., "Herbal medicine for low-back pain."
8. Hoffmann, *Medical Herbalism*, p. 579.
9. Shara and Stohs, "Efficacy and safety of white willow bark extracts."

Chapter 25

1. Jyh-Gang Leu et al., "Epigallocatechin-3-gallate combined with alpha lipoic acid attenuates high glucose-induced receptor for advanced glycation end products (RAGE) expression in human embryonic kidney cells," *Anais da Academia Brasileira de Ciências*, April–June 2013; 85(2): 745–52, www.ncbi.nlm.nih.gov /pubmed/23780308, accessed June 24, 2013.
2. Bob Capelli and Gerald R. Cysewski, *Astaxanthin: Natural Astaxanthin—King of the Carotenoids* (Holualoa, HI: Cyanotech, 2007), p. 19.
3. Ibid., pp. 31–32.
4. Ibid., p. 35.
5. Christiane Staiger, "Comfrey: a clinical overview," *Phytotherapy Research*, October 2012; 26(10): 1441–48, www.ncbi.nlm.nih.gov/pmc/articles/PMC3491633/, accessed February 2, 2020.
6. Ibid.
7. Doug B. Smith and Bert H. Jacobson, "Effect of a blend of comfrey root extract (*Symphytum officinale* L.) and tannic acid creams in the treatment of osteoarthritis of the knee: randomized, placebo-controlled, double-blind, multiclinical trials," *Journal of Chiropractic Medicine*, September 2011; 10(3): 147–56, https:// pubmed.ncbi.nlm.nih.gov/22014903/, accessed March 2, 2020.
8. David J. Fast et al., "*Echinacea purpurea* root extract inhibits TNF release in response to Pam3Csk4 in a phosphatidylinositol-3-kinase dependent manner," *Cellular Immunology*, October 2015; 297(2): 94–99, https://pubmed.ncbi.nlm .nih.gov/26190752/, accessed March 1, 2020.
9. Daniel A. Todd et al., "Ethanolic *Echinacea purpurea* extracts contain a mixture of cytokine-suppressive and cytokine-inducing compounds, including some that originate from endophytic bacteria," *PLOS One*, May 1, 2015; 10(5): e0124276, https://pubmed.ncbi.nlm.nih.gov/25933416/, accessed January 2, 2020.
10. Angela Notarnicola et al., "Comparison of shock wave therapy and nutraceutical composed of *Echinacea angustifolia*, alpha lipoic acid, conjugated linoleic acid, and quercetin (perinerv) in patients with carpal tunnel syndrome," *International Journal of Immunopathology and Pharmacology*, June 2015; 28(2): 256–62, https://pubmed.ncbi.nlm.nih.gov/25953494/, accessed March 1, 2020.
11. Phyllis A. Balch and James F. Balch, *Prescription for Nutritional Healing*, 3rd ed. (New York: Avery, 2000), p. 72.
12. "Guggul," www.webmd.com/vitamins/ai/ingredientmono-591/guggul, accessed November 27, 2020.
13. Steven Horne, "Guggul and myrrh gum (*Commiphora mukul* and *C. myrrha*)," http://treelite.com/articles/articles/guggul-and-myrrh-gum-%28commiphora -mukul-and-c-myrrha%29.html, accessed March 1, 2020.
14. Ibid.
15. "Guggul," https://www.webmd.com/vitamins/ai/ingredientmono-591/guggul, accessed December 1, 2020.
16. Ye Elaine Wang et al., "Association of dietary fatty acid intake with glaucoma in the United States," *JAMA Ophthalmology*, February 1, 2018; 136(2): 141–47, https://pubmed.ncbi.nlm.nih.gov/29270632/, accessed March 1, 2020.
17. Benjamin P. Casella, "Diet change may affect glaucoma risk," *Optometry Times*, April 17, 2018, www.optometrytimes.com/view/diet-change-may-affect -glaucoma-risk, accessed March 3, 2020.

18. J. M. Kremer et al., "Dietary fish oil and olive oil supplementation in patients with rheumatoid arthritis. Clinical and immunological effects," *Arthritis and Rheumatism*, June 1990; 33(6): 810–20, https://pubmed.ncbi.nlm.nih.gov/2363736/, accessed March 1, 2020.

Chapter 26

1. "Profiling food consumption in America," chap. 2 in *Agriculture Fact Book*, US Department of Agriculture, www.usda.gov/factbook/chapter2.pdf, https://www.dhhs.nh.gov/dphs/nhp/documents/sugar.pdf, accessed December 1, 2020.

2. Nancy Appleton, *Lick the Sugar Habit: Sugar Addiction Upsets Your Whole Body Chemistry* (New York: Avery, 1988).

3. Melissa Conrad Stöppler, "Insulin resistance," www.medicinenet.com/insulin_resistance/article.htm, March 12, 2020.

4. Honor Whiteman, "Broccoli sprout extract may help to treat type 2 diabetes," www.medicalnewstoday.com/articles/317917, accessed January 7, 2020.

5. Patrice D. Cani et al., "Involvement of gut microbiota in the development of low-grade inflammation and type-2 diabetes associated with obesity," *Gut Microbes*, July–August 2012; 3(4): 279–88, https://pubmed.ncbi.nlm.nih.gov/22572877/, accessed January 24, 2020.

6. Sonal Gupta Jain et al., "Effect of oral cinnamon intervention on metabolic profile and body composition of Asian Indians with metabolic syndrome: a randomized, double-blind control trial," *Lipids in Health and Disease*, June 12, 2017; 16(1): 113, https://pubmed.ncbi.nlm.nih.gov/28606084/, accessed January 19, 2020.

7. Leslie Ridgeway, "High fructose corn syrup linked to diabetes," https://news.usc.edu/44415/high-fructose-corn-syrup-linked-to-diabetes/, accessed January 29, 2020.

8. Mark Hyman, "5 reasons high fructose corn syrup will kill you," https://drhyman.com/blog/2011/05/13/5-reasons-high-fructose-corn-syrup-will-kill-you/, accessed February 1, 2020.

9. Brian Hoffmann et al., "The influence of sugar and artificial sweeteners on vascular health during the onset and progression of diabetes," Experimental Biology 2018 conference, San Diego, CA, April 22, 2018, https://plan.core-apps.com/eb2018/abstract/382e0c7eb95d6e76976fbc663612d58a, accessed January 27, 2020.

10. Karol Rycerz and Jadwiga Elżbieta Jaworska-Adamu, "Effects of aspartame metabolites on astrocytes and neurons," *Folia Neuropathologica*, 2013; 51(1): 10–17, https://pubmed.ncbi.nlm.nih.gov/23553132/, accessed January 28, 2020.

11. Catharine Paddock, "Study shows dopamine may play role in chronic pain," www.medicalnewstoday.com/articles/293713, accessed January 28, 2020. Stephania Paredes et al., "An association of serotonin with pain disorders and its modulation by estrogens," *International Journal of Molecular Sciences*, November 2019; 20(22): 5729, www.ncbi.nlm.nih.gov/pmc/articles/PMC6888666/, accessed January 28, 2020.

12. Arbind Kumar Choudhary and Etheresia Pretorius, "Revisiting the safety of aspartame," *Nutrition Reviews*, September 1, 2017; 75(9): 718–30, https://pubmed.ncbi.nlm.nih.gov/28938797/, accessed January 11, 2020.

13. Jotham Suez et al., "Artificial sweeteners induce glucose intolerance by altering the gut microbiota," *Nature*, October 9, 2014; 514(7521): 181–86, https://pubmed.ncbi.nlm.nih.gov/25231862/, accessed January 12, 2020.
14. Rajendrakumar M. Patel. et al., "Popular sweetener sucralose as a migraine trigger," *Headache: The Journal of Head and Face Pain*, August 22, 2006; 46(8), 1303–4, https://headachejournal.onlinelibrary.wiley.com/doi/full/10.1111/j.1526-4610.2006.00543_1.x, accessed January 8, 2020.
15. Sumit Bhattacharyya et al., "Exposure to common food additive carrageenan alone leads to fasting hyperglycemia and in combination with high fat diet exacerbates glucose intolerance and hyperlipidemia without effect on weight," *Journal of Diabetes Research*, 2015; 2015: 513429, https://pubmed.ncbi.nlm.nih.gov/25883986/, accessed January 17, 2020.
16. Sumit Bhattacharyya et al., "Carrageenan-induced colonic inflammation is reduced in Bcl10 null mice and increase in IL-10-deficient mice," *Mediators of Inflammation*, 2013; 2013: 397642, https://pubmed.ncbi.nlm.nih.gov/23766559/, accessed January 12, 2020.
17. "Shopping guide to avoiding organic foods with carrageenan," www.cornucopia.org/2012/05/shopping-guide-to-avoiding-organic-foods-with-carrageenan/, accessed February 1, 2020.
18. Sona Skrovankova et al., "Bioactive compounds and antioxidant activity in different types of berries," *International Journal of Molecular Sciences*, October 16, 2015; 16(10): 24673–706, https://pubmed.ncbi.nlm.nih.gov/26501271/, accessed January 13, 2020.
19. Rachel L. Galli et al., "Blueberry supplemental diet reverses age-related decline in hippocampal HSP70 neuroprotection," *Neurobiology of Aging*, February 2006; 27(2): 344–50, https://pubmed.ncbi.nlm.nih.gov/15869824/, accessed January 21, 2020.
20. Leonardo Coelho Rabello Lima et al., "Consumption of cherries as a strategy to attenuate exercise-induced muscle damage and inflammation in humans," *Nutrición Hospitalaria*, November 1, 2015; 32(5): 1885–93, https://pubmed.ncbi.nlm.nih.gov/26545642/, accessed January 22, 2020.
21. Lukas Schwingshakl et al., "Effects of olive oil on markers of inflammation and endothelial function—a systematic review and meta-analysis," *Nutrients*, September 11, 2015; 7(9): 7651–75, https://pubmed.ncbi.nlm.nih.gov/26378571/, accessed January 23, 2020.
22. Lisa Parkinson and Russell Keast, "Oleocanthal, a phenolic derived from virgin olive oil: a review of the beneficial effects on inflammatory disease," *International Journal of Molecular Science*, July 2014; 14(7); 12323–24, www.ncbi.nlm.nih.gov/pmc/articles/PMC4139846/, accessed January 24, 2020.
23. Salahuddin Ahmed et al., "*Punica granatum* L. extract inhibits IL-1β-induced expression of matrix metalloproteinases by inhibiting the activation of MAP kinases and NF-κB in human chondrocytes in vitro," *Journal of Nutrition*, September 2005; 135(9): 2096–2102, www.ncbi.nlm.nih.gov/pmc/articles/PMC1315308/pdf/nihms3610.pdf?tool=pmcentrez, accessed January 23, 2020.
24. A. T. Fahim et al., "Effect of pumpkin-seed oil on the level of free radical scavengers induced during adjuvant-arthritis in rats," *Pharmacological Research*, January 1995; 31(1): 73–79, https://pubmed.ncbi.nlm.nih.gov/7784309/, accessed January 11, 2020.

25. Jace Schell et al., "Strawberries improve pain and inflammation in obese adults with radiographic evidence of knee osteoarthritis," *Nutrients*, August 28, 2017; 9(9): 949, https://pubmed.ncbi.nlm.nih.gov/28846633/, accessed January 24, 2020.

26. Arthritis Foundation, "The Emotion-Pain Connection," www.arthritis.org /health-wellness/healthy-living/emotional-well-being/emotional-self-care/the -emotion-pain-connection, accessed March 11, 2020.

27. Mark A. Lumley et al., "Pain and emotion: a biopsychosocial review of recent research," *Journal of Clinical Psychology*, September 2011; 67(9): 942–68, www .ncbi.nlm.nih.gov/pmc/articles/PMC3152687/, accessed January 27, 2020.

28. Gregory N. Bratman et al., "Nature experience reduces rumination and subgenual prefrontal cortex activation," *PNAS* (*Proceedings of the National Academy of Sciences of the United States of America*), July 14, 2015; 112(28): 8567–72, www .pnas.org/content/112/28/8567.abstract, accessed February 7, 2020.

29. Mark S. Taylor et al., "Research note: urban street tree density and antidepressant prescription rates—a cross-sectional study of London, UK," *Landscape and Urban Planning*, April 2015; 136: 174–79, www.sciencedirect.com/science/article /pii/S0169204614002941, accessed February 6, 2020.

30. Daniel Steffens et al., "Prevention of low back pain: a systematic review and meta-analysis," *JAMA Internal Medicine*, February 2016; 176(2): 199–208, https://pubmed.ncbi.nlm.nih.gov/26752509/, accessed January 12, 2020.

31. Geun Hee Seol et al., "Antidepressant-like effect of *Salvia sclarea* is explained by modulation of dopamine activities in rats," *Journal of Ethnopharmacology*, July 6, 2010; 130(1): 187–90, https://pubmed.ncbi.nlm.nih.gov/20441789/, accessed February 7, 2020.

32. Arieh Moussaieff et al., "Incensole acetate reduces depressive-like behavior and modulates hippocampal BDNF and CRF expression of submissive animals," *Journal of Psychopharmacology*, December 2012; 26(12): 1584–93, https://pubmed .ncbi.nlm.nih.gov/23015543/, accessed February 7, 2020.

33. Razieh Shirzadegan et al., "Effects of geranium aroma on anxiety among patients with acute myocardial infarction: a triple-blind randomized clinical trial," *Complementary Therapies in Clinical Practice*, November 2017; 29: 201–6, www.ncbi .nlm.nih.gov/pubmed/29122262, accessed November 27, 2020.

34. Masoud Nikfarjam et al., "The effects of *Lavandula angustifolia* Mill infusion on depression in patients using citalopram: a comparison study," *Iranian Red Crescent Medical Journal*, August 2013; 15(8): 734–39, https://pubmed.ncbi.nlm.nih .gov/24578844/, accessed February 7, 2020.

35. Víctor López et al., "Exploring pharmacological mechanisms of lavender (*Lavandula angustifolia*) essential oil on central nervous system targets," *Frontiers in Pharmacology*, May 19, 2017; 8: 280, https://pubmed.ncbi.nlm.nih .gov/28579958/, accessed February 7, 2020.

36. Migiwa Komiya et al., "Lemon oil vapor causes an anti-stress effect via modulating the 5-HT and DA activities in mice," *Behavioural Brain Research*, September 25, 2006; 172(2): 240–9, https://pubmed.ncbi.nlm.nih.gov/16780969/, accessed February 7, 2020.

37. Daniele G. Machado et al., "*Rosmarinus officinalis* L. hydroalcoholic extract, similar to fluoxetine, reverses depressive-like behavior without altering learning deficit in olfactory bulbectomized mice," *Journal of Ethnopharmacology*, August 30,

2012; 143(1): 158–69, https://pubmed.ncbi.nlm.nih.gov/22721880/, accessed February 8, 2020.

38. J. Lehrner et al., "Ambient odor of orange in a dental office reduces anxiety and improves mood in female patients," *Physiology & Behavior*, October 1–15, 2000; 71(1–2): 83–86, www.ncbi.nlm.nih.gov/pubmed/11134689, accessed November 27, 2020.

39. Nan Zhang et al., "*Cananga odorata* essential oil reverses the anxiety induced by 1-(3-chlorophenyl) piperazine through regulating the MAPK pathway and serotonin system in mice," *Journal of Ethnopharmacology*, June 12, 2018; 219: 23–30, www.sciencedirect.com/science/article/pii/S0378874117303483?via%3Dihub, accessed November 27, 2020.

INDEX

ABOUT THE AUTHOR

Michelle Schoffro Cook, PhD, DNM, RNCP

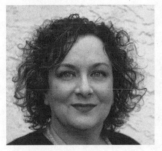

Michelle Schoffro Cook is an international best-selling and twenty-four-time book author whose works include *The Essential Oils Healing Deck, Be Your Own Herbalist, 60 Seconds to Slim, The Ultimate pH Solution*, and *The Cultured Cook*. She is a board-certified doctor of natural medicine, registered nutritionist, certified herbalist, and aromatherapist.

Her books are distributed worldwide and have been translated into many languages, including Greek, Chinese, Indonesian, Russian, Spanish, and Thai.

Her blogs and articles have been featured in or on Care2.com, Yahoo!, *Mother Earth Living, Fermentation, Huffington Post*, and *alive* magazine. Cook's work has been featured in or on *Woman's World* magazine, *First for Women* magazine, WebMD, Reviews.com, *Closer Weekly*, the *Vancouver Sun*, Thrive Global, *Hello!* magazine, *Vegetarian Times, Glow*, the *Ottawa Citizen*, the *Vancouver Sun*, the *Calgary Herald*, and many other publications and sites.

She is the publisher of the popular free health e-newsletter *World's Healthiest News*, which reaches over ten thousand readers in over a hundred countries worldwide. Discover how to maximize the healing power of essential oils by joining Dr. Cook's Medical Aromatherapy team, available through her website at DrMichelleCook.com/Opportunity.

Learn more about her work at DrMichelleCook.com and at Lost Orchard.org.

Connect with Michelle on Instagram: DrMichelleCook; Facebook: DrMichelleCook and DrSchoffroCook; and Twitter: mschoffrocook.